AN INTRODUCTION TO CONCEPTS OF NUTRITION:
A Participant Workbook

AN INTRODUCTION TO CONCEPTS OF NUTRITION:
A Participant Workbook

A Facilitated Course Designed for Further
Education and Entry Level Higher Education /
Adult and Community Learning

Anja Morris-Paxton

To order additional copies of this book, contact:
Xlibris
800-056-3182
www.Xlibrispublishing.co.uk
Orders@Xlibrispublishing.co.uk
791485

BASIC INFORMATION ABOUT
THIS PROGRAMME

Programme Title	:	An Introduction to Concepts of Nutrition
Programme Level	:	Further and Foundational Higher Education
		Adult and Community Learning (ACL)
Hours Required	:	36 hours facilitated learning
Pre-requisite Abilities	:	Grade 12
		Basic application of number and the ability to speak read and write, in the English language medium

CONTENTS

LEARNING SESSION THREE: PROTEIN - WHAT IT IS AND THE SPECIAL ROLE IT HAS IN OUR HEALTH 63

LEARNING SESSION FOUR: THE FAT-SOLUBLE VITAMINS...85

PROGRAMME REVIEWER

Malcolm J Dedman

Malcolm Dedman graduated from Brunel University with an Honours Degree in Technology (Applied Physics) and worked for more than 20 years in the sound technology and engineering industry, where he was responsible for several research and development projects. Malcolm has always had a keen interest in both music and health and later graduated with distinction from Thames Valley University with a Masters in Music Composition. Malcolm brings with him skills in reviewing, proofing and editing research reports and technical manuals and has reviewed the material in this course for literary content, accuracy, and presentation. In addition, he has taken the stance of a programme participant in his critique of the appropriateness and usefulness of the content.

REVIEW OF THE INTRODUCTION TO CONCEPTS OF NUTRITION

Topics such as nutrition, health management, disease prevention and weight-related disorders are all highly emotive subjects, there being vast amounts of literature available. Faced with so much information, the majority of us finds wading through it all is not only time-consuming but is also very confusing as the reader is presented with often conflicting and sometimes controversial information. In this programme, Dr Morris-Paxton takes the mystery out of these topics, as her starting point is both medical and scientific, drawing not only from the latest research but also from her vast knowledge of the areas she covers.

It may not be essential for all participants to understand the detailed background material in the programme fully, as the information is given to show how certain conclusions are reached; but it is the knowledge of these conclusions that will benefit the participant in understanding what foods do for them. In particular, knowledge will be gained about which foods, drinks, vitamins, nutrients, etc. assist our health and those that compromise it. The detailed background material is included, along with many references, to show the interested participant how these conclusions are derived. In addition, Dr Morris-Paxton does not take the approach of telling the participants what they must or must not eat but, instead, by means of interesting and enjoyable exercises, quizzes and discussion sessions, help them to decide for themselves, drawing from their cultural influences and personal tastes.

To say that this subject should be taught in schools as a mandatory part of the National Curriculum is an understatement. The knowledge gained from this programme is essential to everyone, enabling individuals to choose their own paths to a healthier existence, reducing their chances of a major illness, maximising their ability to manage their weight and nutritional programme, all without sacrificing the pleasures gained from eating. Time is also devoted to helping the participants to make changes to their eating habits, where necessary; to plan menus for themselves and their families; as well as giving guidance for keeping to a realistic budget. This programme is not only enjoyable and informative but is also a 'must' for everyone.

Malcolm Dedman, B Tech (Hons), MMus

INTRODUCTION

Welcome

Welcome to 'An Introduction to the Concepts of Nutrition'. The aim of this programme is to facilitate a unique learning environment in which you can develop the underpinning knowledge and skills required for the prevention of ill-health through appropriate nutritional means. The material has been developed where possible from academically accepted reference books and peer-reviewed research papers, as well as the expertise and experience of the author. This means that all the scientific facts that we have given can be verified. You will find the references for these at the end of each learning session in this workbook.

The principles of both nutrition and the methods applied to provide new knowledge and understanding, in this programme are holistic. This means that we have considered the psychological, social, emotional and affective context in which people nourish themselves and others in their family and surroundings. As this programme is facilitated, you will be guided by the facilitator throughout your learning.

The nature of facilitated learning programmes is that you are encouraged to make your own decisions and to help one another as a group. The nature of your participation is for you to gain the knowledge, understanding and skills that you feel can benefit you the most. Your facilitator will help you make decisions that are appropriate to your own circumstances but will not tell you what to do with your life!

All the learning sessions are of equal length and will be conducted in two parts with most of the new knowledge being given in the first half of the session, whilst you are fresh. Your facilitator will lead the sessions and help you as a group with the learning together activities and the discussions in the second part of each session. All the notes are provided for you in this workbook as are the quick quizzes, learning together activities and discussion topics. There is space for you to write and make your own notes so that you have all your work for this programme together in one place.

Creating this programme has been an interesting and enjoyable experience. It is my hope that the result is an equally interesting and enjoyable venture into the world of nutrition for you as a participant.

A A Morris-Paxton

OVERVIEW OF THE PROGRAMME

The concepts of nutrition encompass two kinds of knowledge and ability; the first is a knowledge and understanding of the individual nutrients that we need as human beings to work, learn, socialise and exercise at our best. We need to understand what they are, what they do and what happens if we do not have these nutrients. The second is the ability to use these nutrients together, to understand which foods and substances they come from and what to do with these foods and substances so that we get all of the nutrients we need in the amounts that we need them.

This programme looks at nutrition from a holistic point of view in that it not only gives the facts about the nutrients we need but also looks at what to do with our new-found knowledge and understanding. The programme encompasses twelve facilitated learning sessions the first eight of which look at the background knowledge of nutrients. In sessions nine to twelve we review our application of knowledge about nutrients and the foods that contain them and more specifically how we apply nutrition in our own environment, given our own resources with respect to time, facilities and budget.

Aims of the Programme

1. To acquire knowledge of what the essential nutrients are and in which foods and substances they are to be found, the basis of how the body utilises nutrients, and what happens if one is deficient in particular nutrients.
2. To develop the ability to recognise which foods contain which nutrients and how best to consume these foods so that one obtains the maximum nutritional benefit from them.
3. To develop the ability and confidence to prevent problems that arise from incorrect eating habits and to apply nutritional solutions in the context of one's own environment.
4. To appraise the tools that can be used to plan a diet, produce menus and build one's own recipe portfolio for use within one's own environment.

Learning Outcomes

When you have completed this programme, you should be able to:

1. Demonstrate knowledge of what the essential nutrients are and, in which foods and substances they are found.
2. Demonstrate an understanding of the basis of how the body utilises nutrients and what happens if one is deficient in particular nutrients.
3. Demonstrate a knowledge of which foods contain which nutrients and how these foods are best consumed so that one obtains the maximum nutritional benefit from them.
4. Have the ability and the confidence to prevent problems in one's own environment that arise from incorrect eating habits.
5. Apply nutritional solutions to potential problems in the context of one's own environment.
6. Use given tools to plan diet, menus and build a recipe portfolio for one's own personal use.

The Acquisition of Other Skills

In addition to the above, there are other skills that we anticipate you will acquire and / or develop successfully because of your participation in this course. This will apply if you attend each of the learning sessions, follow the leadership and direction of your course facilitator and complete all the class activities. Such skills include:

Communication Skills:

- Taking part in discussions about straightforward subjects, by:
  - Providing information that is relevant to the subject and purpose of the discussion
  - Speaking clearly in a way that suits the situation
  - Listening and responding appropriately to what others say

- Reading and identifying the main points and ideas from visual presentations and written notes about the programme subject (s) by:
  - Reading material that has been provided
  - Identifying the main points and ideas accurately in this material
  - Using the information to suit your purpose

Skills in the application of number:

- Obtaining the information you need to meet the purpose of your task by:
  - Identifying suitable calculations to get the results you need
  - Carrying out calculations, using whole numbers, simple decimals, fractions and percentages
  - Checking with someone that your results make sense
  - Interpreting the results of your calculations
  - Explaining your findings clearly

Skills in working with others:

- Work closely with one or more other people to meet given objectives and demonstrate that you can understand what needs to be done to achieve these objectives by:
  - Checking that you clearly understand the objectives you have been given for working together by discussing them with others
  - Identifying what needs to be done to achieve these objectives and suggest ways in which you could help
  - Making sure that you are clear about your responsibilities and working arrangements
  - Saying how you have got on and suggest ways of improving how you work with others
- Carry out tasks to meet your responsibilities by:
  - Working safely and accurately following the working methods you have been given

- Asking for help and offering support to others, when appropriate
- Identify what has gone well in working with others
- Reporting any difficulties in meeting your responsibilities and say what you did about them
- Suggest ways of improving work with others to help achieve the objectives

Skills in Improving Your Own Learning and Performance

- Work together with someone to show that you can:
  - Understand the short-term targets they have been given and plan how these will be met
  - Make sure targets clearly show what you want to achieve
  - Identify clear action points and deadlines for each target
  - Identify how to get the support you need and the arrangements for reviewing your progress
- Follow a plan to meet targets and improve performance by:
  - Working through your action points to complete tasks on time
  - Use support given by others to help you meet targets
  - Use different ways of learning suggested by your facilitator, and make changes, when needed, to improve your performance
- Review your own progress and achievements by:
  - Saying what you learned and how you learned, including what has gone well and what has gone less well
  - Identifying targets you have met and your achievements
  - Checking what you need to do to improve your performance

Problem Solving Skills

- Identifying one's own problem(s) and work closely with someone to find and implement a solution by showing that you can:
  - Understand the problem and identify options for solving it

- Identify different ways of tackling the problem
- Decide, with help, which options are most likely to be successful
- Try out options using support and advice given by others
- Confirm with an appropriate person the option you will use for solving the problem
- Plan how to carry out this option
- Follow through your plan, making use of advice and support given by others
- Check if the problem has been solved by appraising the results
- Identify ways of improving your approach to problem-solving

MANAGING YOUR LEARNING EXPERIENCE

As part of your personal and professional development, you will be encouraged to identify problems that you or others may be experiencing that are related to your or their nutritional intake. You will be encouraged, as part of this programme, to apply your new knowledge and understanding to finding and implementing solutions to these problems. You will have the support of your facilitator and the other participants in your learning group, and you may find the 'learning together' sessions and the 'discussion' sessions helpful in this respect.

To gain maximum benefit from this programme, meet the learning outcomes and develop personal skills there are some expectations that participants will be required to meet. These are:

- To attend each learning session
- To be on time for each learning session ready to begin when the session is scheduled to start.
- To remain present throughout each learning session until it has ended
- To complete the 'quick quizzes' as best you can and participate fully in the learning together activities.
- To participate in the discussions
- To follow the guidance of your facilitator

ASSESSMENT OF YOUR LEARNING

The assessment of your learning in this workbook is continuous and formative; there will however be some form of summative course assessment set by your facilitator which may include tests, examinations or a portfolio of work. Achievement rests solely on yourself with the support of your facilitator and the other participants in your programme. There are three types of formative learning activities in each session. Quick quizzes are given throughout the section on acquiring new knowledge, and you may complete these by yourself, in groups or as a class. There are, in addition, some fun group learning activities in which you will participate. These are done in the second half of each session and are designed to help you apply the new knowledge and understanding that you have gained. Your facilitator will give you feedback on how you have completed your learning activities; however, you will also be asked to ascertain for yourself how much you have achieved during the sessions. Towards the end of the session, there will be a discussion topic involving all the participants together as a group and will be led by the facilitator. He or she will give feedback on your participation and summarise the consensus of opinion.

On completion of the course, if you have attended all of the sessions and have participated as fully as possible in the learning together activities and the discussions, you will have met the learning outcomes for this programme.

THE LEARNING SESSIONS

Learning Session One: The Importance of Nutrition and an Introduction to the Essential Nutrients

This session covers the importance of nutrition, the role that malnutrition and nutritional imbalances play in the generation of chronic disease and the rate of non-recovery from communicable diseases. It highlights how good nutrition can be a major preventative measure against future ill health and can aid in recovery and recuperation from current ill-health and recent surgical intervention. In addition, the essential nutrients are highlighted, and we discover together what they are, why they are essential to our long-term survival and health and where they come from.

Learning Session Two: Carbohydrates and Fats, What They Are and What They Do

This session looks at the elements that make up the basic structure of carbohydrates and fats, how these two substances are similar and what makes them different. We discover how carbohydrates give us the bulk of our energy and what the best sources of carbohydrates are. We also look at the damage done by refined carbohydrates and why we need to avoid having too many of these. In addition, we look at what the essential fats are and what they do, why we need some kinds of fat for good health and why other kinds may produce problems over the long term.

Learning Session Three: Protein, What It Is and the Special Role It Has in Our Health

This session discusses the basic building blocks of protein, the amino acids, and looks at which ones are essential to us. We also take a look at the protein-rich foods and, more essentially, the net usable protein that we obtain from these foods. You might find that there are possibly some surprises for you in this respect. We then move on to the combining of protein-rich and carbohydrate-rich foods and the controversy surrounding this in some schools of thought.

Learning Session Four: The Fat-Soluble Vitamins

In this session we look at four of the vitamins, in particular, A, D E, and K. We discover together what these vitamins do individually and working in synergy with one another. These vitamins are fat soluble and the only ones that the body is capable of storing in any significant amounts. We discuss the advantages and disadvantages of this property and how to obtain enough to benefit ourselves without the problems of accumulating too much.

Learning Session Five: The Water-Soluble Vitamins

Now we come to the rest of the vitamins, those that are water soluble and that the body cannot store. These are the B-complex vitamins and Vitamin C, which works together with other substances that we cannot really separate it from, the bioflavonoids. We discover what they do and how important they are to many aspects of our health. We look at normal requirements for these and the circumstances where one may require a little more than the average daily intake.

Learning Session Six: The Minerals

In this session, we look at the often-forgotten items in our nutritional intake, the minerals. Those we need a fair amount of are the macronutrients, and those we require in very small amounts are micronutrients. All, however, are vital to our health and we look at what happens when we have an imbalance of these substances and how to avoid this, both by obtaining a variety of foods and by using mineral-rich foods in the correct amounts.

Learning Session Seven: Fibre and Phytonutrients

The two other frequently forgotten items of nutrition are fibre and the phytonutrients. Fibre comes in insoluble and soluble forms and constitutes a part of unprocessed foods of vegetable origin. We look at the role of fibre and how to avoid the problems that occur when not enough of this substance is taken in. In addition, we discover the often-overlooked phytonutrients. Substances of value that are often found in herbs spices and cooking ingredients are the phytonutrients. We often miss out on the benefits of these due to the way in which we prepare food and cultural preferences for a particular way of cooking. We look at the benefits of these substances and how we can incorporate them into our diet.

<u>Learning Session Eight: The Essential Elements</u>

Here we look at the elements we need to survive, what they are and why they are essential and, most importantly, what they have to do with a programme on nutrition! Water, air and sunlight are essential to all growth whether that of plants, animals or human beings. We discover why and how these are important to human life, and the development and the utilisation of all the other nutrients. We look at the issue of both quantity of these substances and quality, at a balanced intake where we gain the maximum benefit with the minimum damage.

<u>Learning Session Nine: Energy, Body Composition and Weight</u>

In this session, we discover what it is that our body does with the food we eat, how energy is generated in the body's cells and what happens to the excess we take in. We look at the issue of calories, what they are, what they do and how important or unimportant the actual calorie count of food might be. We discover the difference between body weight and body composition and how we can tell what is best for us as an individual.

<u>Learning Session Ten: Putting the Nutrients Together</u>

We discover in this session the tools we can use to put our new-found knowledge and understanding together. We explore the use of various designs of the food pyramids, food exchange lists, and the advantages and considerations of these. We also explore the author's own tool; 'The Colour Wheel' and how this can be customised for one's own personal needs and used together with other tools. We look at portions, sizes and what constitutes an item of food or a food exchange. The timing of foods, meals and snacks is looked at. In addition, we gain an understanding of why breakfast is so important and how to get over the problem of early morning lack of appetite.

Learning Session Eleven: Building Recipes

Here we look at what we can do with your old recipes, changing ingredients, changing cooking methods and improving on what you already have. We also look at how you can build new nutritious recipes from the basis of the knowledge you have now acquired and using the tools from the previous session. We discover how we can create our own dietary plan, one that we can enjoy as opposed to one that has been designed by someone else to their own tastes.

Learning Session Twelve: Menu Planning and Shopping Lists

Putting together menu plans is the focus of this session. We look at planning menus from your own recipes that fit in with your own nutritional programme. We also look at what to do about family menus and menus that will suit both you and others that you might be caring and cooking for. We look at seasonal recipes and menus and how to create shopping lists to match these. We look at the constraints one might have such as time and equipment as well as convenience and distance from the places you shop. Finally, we look at the advantages and hazards of shopping online, how to create standard food orders and plan to a budget.

LEARNING SESSION ONE: THE IMPORTANCE OF NUTRITION AND AN INTRODUCTION TO THE ESSENTIAL NUTRIENTS

Introduction

Nutrition is currently a hot topic and has been the subject of TV programmes, radio talks, chat shows and even a movie! It has hit the media in magazine articles, books and celebrity diets. However how much do we really know and how do we know that what we are being told is right or not? Knowledge abounds on the internet and in popular fad diet books but what we do with it and how we wade through the plethora of information to find out what we can apply and how requires perhaps a little guidance. This course aims to provide the necessary knowledge you require alongside encouragement and assistance from your programme facilitator.

This first session will look at why nutrition is so important to our health and long-term well-being. We discuss the definition of health as well as the definitions of communicable and chronic diseases. We also look at how undernutrition and malnutrition are defined and the role that malnutrition and nutritional imbalances play in the generation of chronic disease and the rate of recovery from communicable diseases. The session then highlights how good nutrition can be a major preventative measure against future ill health.

Together we then move on to the essential nutrients, and we discover together what they are, why they are essential to our long-term survival and health and where they come from. The session includes the elements which are often forgotten, and why we require these. Later in this session, we come to the learning together section where we will gather into small groups for two learning activities. These should be moderately challenging, but fun and assistance will be available from your facilitator. Finally, we come to the general discussion which is conducted as a whole group. The subject for the discussion today will be 'Malnutrition in Modern Societies'.

THE IMPORTANCE OF NUTRITION IN OUR LIVES

As far back as 1978, the Declaration of Alma-Ata challenged the world to embrace the principles of primary health care as the way to overcome gross health inequalities between and within countries. "Health for all" became the slogan for a movement, in which it was recognised that everybody needs and is entitled to the highest possible standard of health. All countries of the world have pledged to reach the Sustainable Development Goals set by the United Nations in 2015. These include ambitious targets for nutrition and we now have an opportunity to gain the knowledge we need for longer, healthier lives and to lay the foundations for improved health for generations to come [1].

Before we move on to the main subject of this section, let's look first at the whole issue of health and ill-health. Health is not simply the absence of disease or of infirmity but has been defined as *a state of complete physical, mental and social well-being*. The health of any group of people is both a goal in itself and a key development input towards other goals. This is because health contributes crucially to economic and social well-being. More recently, health has not been seen in isolation but in conjunction with human wealth and the lack of health, therefore, is viewed alongside the issue of *human poverty*. This term refers to deprivation of the means to achieve capabilities, for example, physical access to health care in addition to the lack of basic factors that facilitate this achievement such as social access to health care. *Human development* refers to processes that enlarge people's choices to enable them to achieve capabilities, for example, the freedom to choose a healthy lifestyle and the information with which to make a genuinely informed choice about one's lifestyle (such as engaging with this programme). This more complex concept of poverty, wealth and development takes account of the interactive processes that are crucial to the social dynamics of health improvement, significantly, ill-health limits people's ability to earn higher incomes [1].

When we discuss health, we are in fact discussing how not to develop a disease or illness. Two types of disease have been identified; those which are communicable and those which have previously been known as non-communicable diseases, now more often termed chronic diseases.

Communicable diseases are those which are infectious and are spread from person to person, or via other vectors such as infected food, or water. These include:

Measles	SARS
Tuberculosis	HIV
Poliomyelitis	Hepatitis (all kinds)

The previously termed non-communicable diseases are those generated most often through a combination of hereditary tendencies and lifestyle factors, (not necessarily in equal measure) such as:

Cardiovascular Disease	Obesity
Hypertension	Cancers
Type 2 Diabetes	Osteoporosis

It has, however, been argued that these are also 'communicable', not so much as by human contact, but by the person to person transmission of certain social habits and lifestyles. Inappropriate lifestyle is still communicable; however, the vectors (means of spreading disease) are not skin contact or coughing but peer pressure, marketing pressure and family habits that continue from generation to generation. Also, inadequate access to information with which to make informed decisions comes into the equation. We no longer, therefore, refer to these diseases as non-communicable but as chronic disorders most of which are lifestyle and diet-related and in addition preventable [2].

The burden of chronic disorders is increasing, accounting for nearly half of the global burden of disease. While the proportion of burden from chronic diseases in developed countries remains stable at over 80% in adults aged 15 years and over, the proportion in middle-income countries has already exceeded 70%. Surprisingly, almost

50% of the adult disease burden in the high mortality regions of the world is now attributable to chronic diseases. Cardiovascular diseases account for 13% of the disease burden among adults over 15 years of age. Ischaemic heart disease and cerebrovascular disease (stroke) are the two leading causes of mortality and disease burden among older adults (over age 60). In developed countries, ischaemic heart disease and cerebrovascular disease are together responsible for 36% of deaths. The mortality and burden resulting from cardiovascular diseases are rapidly increasing in developing regions as well. Of the 7.1 million cancer deaths estimated to have occurred in 2002, 17% were liver and colon/ rectum cancers which are the third and fourth leading causes of death [1].

All the chronic diseases mentioned previously are preventable, and the main source of prevention is the improvement of healthy eating and physical activity. These are the two goals of the World Health Organisation (WHO) global strategy on diet, physical activity and health [4]. Hypertension is one of the most prevalent problems in Westernised societies, this being the major precursor to stroke. Diet and lifestyle have a substantial impact on the problem of hypertension with being overweight, physical inactivity, high sodium intake and low potassium intake being the main contributors [5]. Upon the conclusion of a four-year research project, the American Institute of Cancer Research concluded that the most appropriate approach to the prevention of cancer by dietary means is the consumption of a whole food diet within the context of existing cultural cuisines [6]. One of the most effective tools of preventative medicine is nutrition education and intervention. Changing the eating habits of a group of people would cut the figures for heart disease, diabetes and some of the preventable cancers along with the misery that comes with them. Many chronic diseases are not only preventable but, if caught in time, can be dealt with solely with a change in diet. Unfortunately, it sometimes takes a crisis in a person's life for them to begin looking at ways to help themselves out of a chronic ill-health problem and to look at ways to prevent further degeneration [7].

Under-nutrition is defined as insufficient nutrients due to inadequate food intake or inadequate assimilation of food (due to illness or gastrointestinal disorders), whereas malnutrition is due to an unbalanced intake of nutrients [3]. These are not necessarily mutually exclusive. That means that although one can be undernourished, one may or may not have the correct balance of nutrients. In the case of malnutrition, one may be undernourished as well, and the problem is that one is receiving both too little food and too little variety of foods. Traditionally we associate these two disorders with one another, and these two terms have sometimes been used interchangeably. Increasingly in modern times and in developed countries, one finds that there is malnutrition that is simply due to imbalances in food intake and not due to either under-nutrition or necessarily shortages of food, poverty or gastrointestinal problems. Causes of this type of mal-nutrition are that either too little variety is eaten, or foods with low nutritional value are consumed. This occurs for instance when people eat chips (fries) with almost every meal or centre each main meal on meat and potatoes. They have too many calories (which we will come to later) and too few essential nutrients, a scenario which leads to certain types of disorders over the long term.

The science of nutrition has changed over the last few years, and where once a balanced diet was one where one ate adequately enough to avoid nutrient deficiencies, we are now at the stage where good nutrition means consuming an optimum diet for promoting health as well as reducing the risk of diet-related disorders. At the turn of the last century, scientists began to embrace the use of optimum nutrition which focuses on optimising the quality of the diet not only in terms of nutritional content but also in terms of non-nutrients as well as other food properties that favour the maintenance and enhancement of health [8]. The WHO report on the prevention of chronic diseases highlighted lifestyle related disorders that had a strong aetiology of long-term nutritional imbalance. The report also adopted an individualistic approach which encourages each person to make individual and sensible dietary choices [9].

We have now seen how nutrition is central to our health and the mitigation of disease. Before we move on to looking at what the individual nutrients that we need for health are, we will try a little exercise. This is something that we will do together.

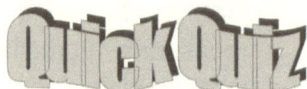

1. In 1978 the Declaration of Alma-Ata resulted in a slogan for a movement, which was:

   Answer: _____

   A. Equality in Health

   B. Health for All

   C. Health for Us

   D. People's Health

2. Health is defined as:

   Answer: _____

   A. The absence of disease

   B. The absence of a disability

   C. Holistic health

   D. Complete physical, mental and social well-being

3. There are two types of diseases:

   Answer: _____

   A. Communicable and chronic diseases

   B. Infectious and contagious diseases

   C. Short term diseases and disabilities

   D. Infectious diseases and genetic diseases

4. The best protection against disease ssuch as cancer is thought to be:

   Answer: _____

   A. Eating as much as you can so as not to be undernourished

   B. Eating as little as you can so as not to consume too many processed foods

   C. Eating a whole food diet made up of one's own cultural foods

   D. Eating a lot from health food shops

5. Optimum nutrition focuses on:

   Answer: _____

   A. The amount of food eaten

   B. The quality of food eaten

   C. Where food comes from

   D When to eat

The Macronutrients: Carbohydrates, Lipids (Fats) and Proteins

An essential nutrient is one which is necessary for our survival. The term 'essential' means two things, firstly that we cannot survive for any meaningful length of time without problems if we do not have this nutrient and secondly, that we cannot manufacture it ourselves. Essential nutrients are those that we must take in from the outside, through foods and fluids in our diet. Essential nutrients are found in all unprocessed, unrefined foods, and they come in two forms; those that we require in bulk are called the *macronutrients,* and those that we require in smaller amounts are termed *micronutrients.* Briefly, we will deal with the macronutrients first. These are the carbohydrates, lipids (fats) and proteins.

Carbohydrates

All organotrophic organisms (trophe is the Greek word for food) ultimately obtain their energy from the sun through a process called *photosynthesis.* This is the process by which plants convert energy from light into chemical energy which is stored within carbon bonds in the molecules that make up the plants tissue. During this process, the plant forms the first stable carbohydrate molecule called a *'triose',* which in turn is converted into glucose and fructose and eventually into sucrose. Sucrose is the basic building block of starch (known as a polysaccharide)[10].

The three chemical elements which form the basis of this process are carbon, oxygen and hydrogen and the resulting sucrose and starches (polysaccharides) are known as carbohydrates. Simple carbohydrates are those which are predominantly made of sucrose fructose and / or glucose, and complex carbohydrates are those which are predominantly made up of starch. Carbohydrates are the body's principal source of energy and the most preferred source of energy for metabolic efficiency, they are found in foods, derived from plants with the exception of very small amounts (lactose) found in milk and dairy products[10].

<u>Lipids</u>

Lipids are the building blocks of fats found in both plant and animal-derived foods. Unlike carbohydrates, these are smaller structures which are insoluble in water. Lipids are very dense and contain 2.25 (two and a quarter) times the energy of carbohydrate. Human beings store fat as energy for future use in times of famine. There are two types of fat in the human body; the most important is *structural fat* (known as 'brown fat') which helps to keep the organs in place and protect the nerves from shock and damage. This type of fat contributes to subcutaneous fat, which acts as insulation, preserving and regulating body temperature. The second type is *adipose tissue* or stored fat. Dietary fats, found in fish, seeds, nuts, whole grains, avocado pears and olives are essential for the digestion, absorption, and transport of fat-soluble vitamins[10]. There are three major groups of lipids:

> Fatty acids
> Triglycerides
> Phospholipids

Fatty acids are found in foods and are either saturated or unsaturated. Saturated fats have single bonds, between their components, are dense or solid at room temperature and are found predominantly in foods of animal origin. Unsaturated fats have some double bonds between their components, are liquid at room temperature and are found mainly in foods of vegetable origin. Such fats are often characterised by the location of these double bonds (characterised by the Greek letter 'ω' – omega) which give them different chemical properties. The three essential fatty acids are[10]:

Linoleic acid	- omega 6
Alpha-linolenic acid	- omega 3
Oleic acid	- omega 9

Triglycerides are formed in the body from three fatty acid molecules and a glycerol molecule; they avoid damage that can be caused by circulating free fatty acids that react readily with other molecules and disrupt the integrity of tissues. Phospholipids are a form of modified triglyceride found in the lining of the intestines where they assist in the binding and transportation of dietary fats and oils[10].

Proteins

In a never-ending 'nitrogen cycle', plants incorporate inorganic nitrogen from nitrogen-fixing bacteria to form *amino acids* which are the building blocks of proteins. Animals (and humans) eat the plants and convert the amino acids to the proteins that they require for growth and repair. Finally, everyone dies, organic molecules are degraded by micro-organisms releasing the nitrogen for re-use by nitrogen-fixing bacteria and so the cycle continues[10].

Proteins are required mainly for growth and repair and are especially necessary during childhood and after illness, injury and surgery. Protein-rich foods are found both in the plant and animal kingdom, the best sources being soy, eggs, fish and combinations of grains and pulses. Amino acids are carbohydrates with an amino group added (NH_2 – containing nitrogen). There are 20 amino acids required by humans, which fall into two groups; essential and non-essential. Essential ones are those that humans cannot make, and we have no option but to obtain them from our diet. Non-essential ones can be made from combinations of the essential amino acids. The essential amino acids are[10]:

Phenylalanine	P
Valine	V
Threonine	T
Tryptophan	T
Isoleucine	I
Methionine	M

Histidine	H
Arginine	A
Lysine	L
Leucine	L

Remember that these are the building blocks of life! One way of doing this is to think of the following mnemonic:

Pvt TIM HALL BUILT THE ARMY A WALL!

We will return to these macronutrients in the second and third learning sessions but first, let's see how much we have learned!

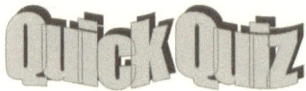

1. How many macronutrients are there?

    Answer: _____

    A. Two

    B. Four

    C. Three

    D. Five

2. The macronutrients are:

    Answer: _____

    A. Molecules containing carbon and molecules containing nitrogen

    B. Fats; Lipids; Starches and Proteins

    C. Carbohydrates; Lipids and Proteins

    D. Sugars; starches; fatty acids; essential amino acids and non-essential amino acids

3. Photosynthesis is the process by Which:

    Answer: _____

    A. Plants give off energy into the atmosphere

    B. Plants convert energy from the sun into chemical energy

    C. Plants process nitrogen from the soil

    D. Sunlight breaks down plant matter

4. The essential fatty acids are:

    Answer: _____

A. Linoleic; alpha linolenic and oleic acids

B. Triglycerids, phospholipids and glycerol

C. Structural fats and non-structural fats

D. Saturated fats and unsaturated fats

The Micronutrients: Vitamins and Minerals

The *micronutrients* are those that are essential to our health and well-being, but we need them in small amounts. They are found within the carbohydrate, lipid and protein-rich foods that produce energy. Whilst the basic functions of the macronutrients are to produce energy for both immediate use and storage and to build and repair body tissues; micronutrients function at the cellular level. That is, they come into our systems via food, which is broken down and digested in the stomach and small intestines, from where the micronutrients are extracted and absorbed into the bloodstream to circulate around the body and 'feed' the individual cells which make up the tissues. Micronutrients consist of *vitamins, minerals, phytonutrients and fibre.* Here we will briefly introduce the vitamins which will be covered a little more fully in learning sessions four and five and the minerals which will be covered more fully in learning session six.

Vitamins

It was the discovery of vitamins that led to the birth of the science that we now know as nutrition[11]. Vitamins, which are essential micronutrients, have the following criteria[11]:

- They are organic compounds (contain carbon), but distinct from the macronutrients (carbohydrates, lipids and proteins).
- They are natural components of unprocessed foods, present usually in minute amounts.
- They are not synthesised in the body in any amount that would be considered adequate to meet normal physiological needs – they are therefore essential.
- Insufficiency of these substances causes a specific deficiency syndrome that adversely affects one's health.

There are eighteen vitamins and vitamin-like substances that we require as humans for health. There are two types of vitamins that we will look at; those that are fat soluble and those that are water soluble. The fat-soluble vitamins are passively absorbed from food – that is they need a little help and require to be transported with a dietary lipid. They tend to be found in the lipid portions of the cellular component of the food. Fat-soluble vitamins can be stored in the body to a certain extent, and therefore the body can sustain itself for a short time if these are not taken in on a daily basis [11]. The fat-soluble vitamins are[11]:

- Vitamin A
- Vitamin E
- Vitamin D
- Vitamin K

The water-soluble vitamins are absorbed both by passive and active mechanisms and may be transported by carriers or absorbed directly from the intestines into the bloodstream alone. They are found in the aqueous (or watery) parts of the cells of foods. Unlike fat-soluble vitamins, water-soluble vitamins cannot be stored by the body and, once absorbed, metabolised and used; any excess is flushed out in the urine. This means that they need to be taken in on a daily basis[11]. These are[11]:

- Vitamin C   - Ascorbic Acid
- Vitamin B Complex
  - B1   - Thiamin
  - B2   - Riboflavin
  - B3   - Niacin
  - B5   - Pantothenic Acid
  - B6   - Pyridoxine
  - -   - Folate
  - B12   - Cobalamin
  - -   - Biotin

Vitamins are obtained mainly from fresh vegetables and fruits, as well as whole grains, pulses, nuts, seeds, and eggs. Other vitamin-like substances that are not strictly vitamins but work together with vitamins and have what is termed vitamin-like behaviour in the body include the substances Choline; Carnitine; myo-Inositol; and the

Ubiquinones and Bioflavonoids. These substances occur naturally in most foods, alongside the other vitamins and as long as your diet has a good variety of whole foods, you will most likely not be deficient in these micronutrients[11].

Minerals

The minerals are a large class of micronutrients most of which are essential. They are found in unprocessed foods and exist in the body mainly in the *ionic* (elemental) state. Although we do not need these in any large amounts as we do the bulk nutrients, there are some minerals that we require in a measurable amount on a daily basis, 100 mg or more (examples are magnesium and calcium) which are termed *macrominerals* and some for which the requirement is very small indeed this being 15mg or less (such as iron and zinc), known as *trace elements*. Recently the term *'ultra-trace elements'* has been used to describe those minerals that we require in microgram (µg) quantities each day, (such as selenium and chromium) [12].

Minerals have many essential functions in the body including serving as ions dissolved in water which keep the 'electrical flow' of the body moving. This is essential for heart and muscle function as well as the functioning of the nervous system. In addition, minerals maintain the balance of water inside and outside of the body's cells, and the correct acidic balance of the body. Minerals form components of the body's cells, which is especially vital in the bone structure and, in addition, maintain the activities of enzyme systems [12].

The essential minerals that we require will be expanded upon later in the course however, for the present we will give you the names of the 18 essential minerals that we know that we need. These are [12]:

Calcium	Ca	Fluorine	Fl
Phosphorous	P	Copper	Cu
Magnesium	Mg	Iodine	I

Sodium	Na	Selenium	Se
Potassium	K	Manganese	Mn
Chloride	Cl	Chromium	Ch
Sulphur	S	Molybdenum	Mo
Iron	Fe	Boron	Bo
Zinc	Zn	Cobalt	Co

Research into how the body utilises minerals and our requirements for minerals has lagged a little behind the knowledge we have acquired about the vitamins. However due to recent improvements in analytical chemistry and techniques for analysing the mineral content of both human tissues and foods we are catching up! Although we may not know exactly how much we need of the ultra-trace elements on a daily basis for good health, we have begun to recognise that they are nevertheless necessary and should not be left out[12].

One ongoing problem with minerals is that plant food, supposedly rich in certain minerals, may not contain as much as we would expect if grown in poor quality soil. This is especially bad in countries where poor farming methods are used or where farmers do not have the money to buy good quality fertiliser or the knowledge of good use of their land. This could mean that in poor communities where nutrition is already compromised, things might be made worse when the food that is consumed has less than the expected quantities of nutrients.

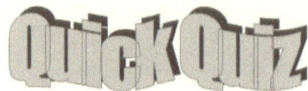

1. The properties of vitamins are that they are:

    Answer: _____

    A. Organic naturally found in foods in small amounts

    B. Inorganic, naturally found in foods in large amounts

    C. Organic, found in whole grains in large amounts

    D. Inorganic and synthesised in the body

2. The properties of minerals are that they are:

    Answer: _____

    A. Organic, found in large amounts in foods and are all essential

    B. Found in inorganic ionic form in foods and most are essential

    C. Organic, not essential but useful for heart and muscle function

    D. All required in large amounts

Other Nutritional Factors: Fibre and Phytonutrients

Although not strictly speaking individual nutrients such as vitamins or minerals, both fibre and phytonutrients have come under the spotlight more due to the adverse effects of their absence from the diet as much as due to their presence.

Dietary Fibre

We will look at the structure of dietary fibre in a little more detail later on in the programme as well as looking at the functions that it has in the body. However, dietary fibre is a component of carbohydrates but, whilst the component of starch comes from the inside of the plant, the component of fibre comes mainly from the structural walls. The cellular structure is slightly different from that of starches. Fibre takes a number of forms, each of which has different properties [13]:

- Cellulose
- Hemicellulose
- Pectins
- Gums

Whilst humans have the enzymes to digest starches we do not have the enzymes to digest dietary fibre. Fibre nevertheless has several essential functions in the gastrointestinal system including[13]:

- Regulation of the absorption of sugars
- Regulation of the absorption of fats
- Encouraging adequate and regular peristalsis in the gastrointestinal tract

Many nutritional scientists blame the incidence of diseases that previously did not exist and are prevalent in Westernised societies on the insufficiency of fibre in the diet. Chronic degenerative diseases such as gout, heart disease, cancer and diabetes can be avoided by increasing dietary fibre and the consumption of unrefined plant foods as part of ones nutritional and lifestyle improvement plan[14]. A study conducted over a fourteen year period positively links an increase in bran from whole grains or added to foods with a decrease in coronary heart disease [15].

<u>Phytonutrients</u>

Phytonutrients are small amounts of substances found in herbs, condiments and other items used with food, but they are not necessarily complete foods. They may have special health-enhancing properties over and above the benefits of the intake of macro-nutrients and baseline amounts of micro-nutrients. There can be two reasons for this:

- The item has a particularly high content of one or more micro-nutrients which have been found beneficial in mitigating or preventing a particular disorder.
- The food has a phytochemical component which has medicinal properties.

Phytonutrients are often used traditionally and can be incorporated easily into cooking; examples are garlic, cayenne pepper, ginger and turmeric. Many herbal teas also contain nutritional substances and have medicinal properties, such as peppermint, rooibos (red bush) and green tea. We will pursue this in a little more depth later in the programme.

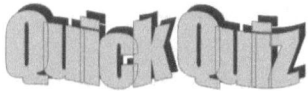

1. Dietary fibre is found in:

   Answer: _____

   A. Stringy meats and chicken

   B. Whole foods of vegetable origin

   C. Processed foods of vegetable origin

   D. A wide variety of plant and animal foods

2. Examples of dietary fibre are

   Answer: _____

   A. Cellulose sucrose and maltose

   B. Lactose, mannose and guar gum

   C. Cellulose, hemicellulose and pectins

   D. Lignin, lycopene and lactose

3. Phytonutrients may have:

   Answer: _____

   A. Nutrient and/or medicinal properties

   B. Chemical and mineral properties

   C. Nutritional and chemical properties

   D. Vitamin and mineral properties

The Essential Elements: Water, Sunlight and Oxygen

If you find yourself feeling fatigued, worn out with no energy and no motivation, the problem may not be your circumstances, or even whether you have eaten or what you have or have not eaten, as much as a deficiency of one of the three most essential requirements to human survival. These are water, sunlight and oxygen.

Water

This is the most abundant inorganic compound in all living systems. It is the criteria by which we define whether life can exist. Without water, there is no possibility of life in any form as we know it. Although one can survive weeks without food, without water one could not survive more than a few days. Nearly all the body's chemical reactions take place in a watery medium, and it is a solvent for minerals and vitamins. In addition, the properties of water allow for it to act as a regulatory mechanism for body temperature[16].

Water is a major component of the body fluids, blood, lymph, and lubricants such as mucous, pleural and pericardial fluids as well as digestive juices. For men, 65% of the body is water, for women 55% of the body is water. Of this, 65% is found inside the cells and 35% outside the cells [17].

Dehydration occurs where there is a decrease in the body's water content whilst the sodium concentration is near normal. The first sign of having insufficient water (dehydration) is not thirst but fatigue. The quality of water and correct fluid intake is so important that the provision of sufficient, safe drinking water has become a major goal of the WHO [18]. Later on in the course, we will look at water and its uses in a little more depth, and we will learn how to calculate one's personal needs for water and how to monitor correctly one's own fluid intake and that of others that we care for.

Sunlight

This is something that one does not normally think of in terms of nutrition or even of health in general; however, most, if not all people feel better on a sunny day.

This is because we need sunlight to produce serotonin, an important neurotransmitter that prevents depression and aids in sleep. In addition, sunlight is also equally as necessary for the production in the body of a substance called cholecalciferol the active form of vitamin D, as dietary intake of vitamin D., it is essential to the health of our bones, the prevention of osteoporosis and osteoarthritis as well as rickets in early childhood [11].

Oxygen

Oxygen is the active element in the gaseous mixture we call air. If a candle is lit it burns in the air but burns more brightly in pure oxygen, and to some extent, this is reflected in our lives and levels of energy[19]. Oxygen is another essential element without which there would be no animal or human life on earth. Oxygen, or rather the quantity and quality is somewhat taken for granted. In fact, there are two issues to be discussed regarding respiration and the intake of air and absorption of oxygen. One is that of lung function and correct breathing for health. The other is that of cellular exchange of oxygen, for the waste product of carbon dioxide and, the nutrients that facilitate this [16]. The air we breathe needs to be of good quality without too many impurities, pollution or dust. How we breathe is also important, and proper breathing is something that few people do, but a technique that can be learnt, to one's advantage [19].

In learning session nine we will look more closely at the elements, the upside of their intake and the downside. We look at how much is enough and how much is too much and the damage that can be caused by an insufficiency or overdose. For now, we will move on to our learning together sessions.

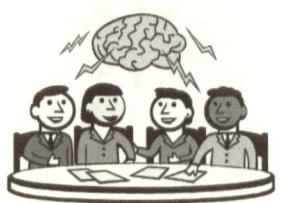

Learning Together
Learning Together

Activity 1.1: Allow yourselves 15 minutes for this activity

Below is a quick crossword puzzle, see if you can solve this between you as a group.

Learning Activity 1.1

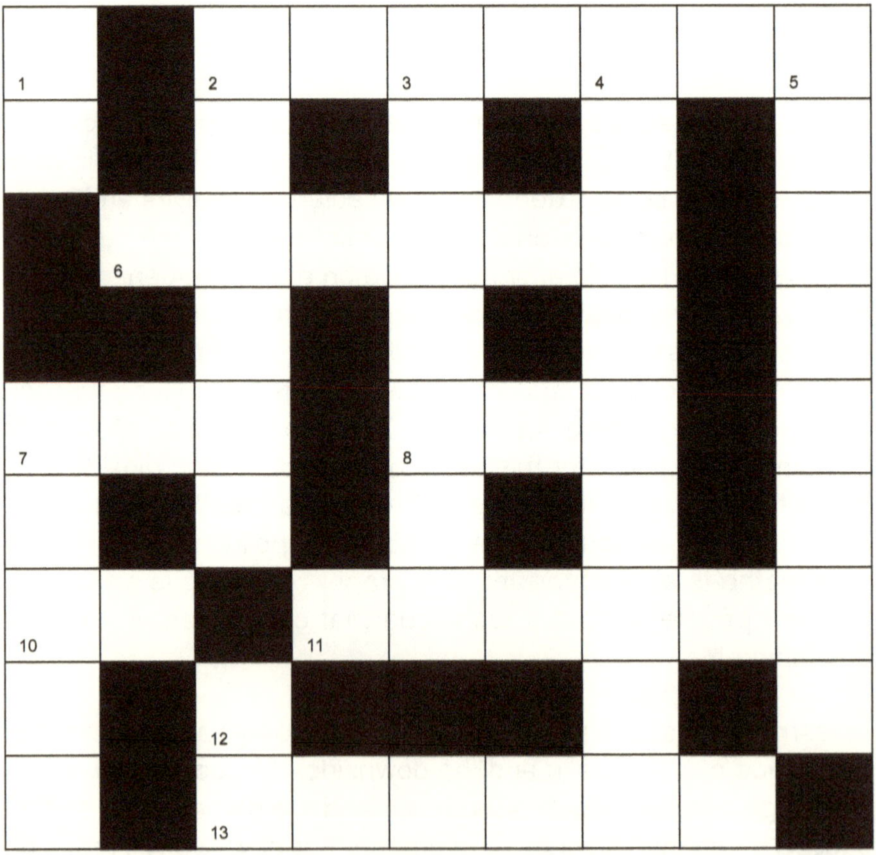

© A. A. Morris-Paxton 2019

Clues:

Across

2. A macronutrient composed of amino acids

6. If you do not control this problem, the result could be hypertension (high blood pressure) and other illnesses

7. A controversial macronutrient which many feel we could do with less of!

8. The elemental minerals are in this form

10. The chemical abbreviation for the mineral boron

11. An essential amino acid

13. An essential mineral and a constituent of vitamin B12

Down

1. Two fat-soluble vitamins that are not synthesised in the body and need to be taken in with food

2. A well-known vegetable rich in starch

3. A major chronic disorder that has recently risen to epidemic proportions

4. The term used for a nutrient that we cannot do without and which we can only acquire through nutrition

5. The element that is in amino acids but not triose or fatty acids

7. The substance which is not a nutrient but nevertheless essential to health and found only in vegetable matter

12. The two water soluble vitamins

Activity 1.2: Allow yourselves 10 minutes for this activity

1.2. a) Count up how many essential micronutrients there are all together and write these down below. Now check to see that you have not left any of them out between you.

1.2. b) How many had you heard of (personally)? How many had no-one in your group heard of before?

1.2. c) Taking your answers into consideration, do you think that you are getting all the nutrients that you require in your diet or do you think that you are inadvertently leaving some of them out?

Write Your Notes Here

Now you should take 5 minutes todiscuss the answers with your facilitator

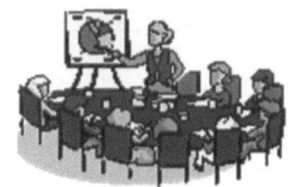

Discussion

Today's Topic for Discussion is: 'MALNUTRITION IN MODERN SOCIETIES'

Westernised, high income, societies appear to have an abundance of food, and more and more people are suffering from the obesity epidemic. Despite this many are becoming ill due to lack of vitamins and minerals and obesity is now co-existent alongside nutritional deficiencies. This is also an emerging problem in middle-income countries such as Southern African and South American countries, where overweight exists alongside nutritional deficiency.

Some questions to think about:

- Are people, in general, eating too much overall or just too much of the wrong foods and not enough of the more nutritious items?
- As a group, do you think that this is generally a big problem, or do you think that the problem is overemphasised by the media and the government?
- Alternatively, do you think the problem is bigger than we thought and the focus of attention on it has come a little too late?
- If you think there is a problem in this area what could you suggest as solutions?

You Might Wish to Write Some Notes Here

References

1. United Nations. United Nations Sustainable Development Goals: United Nations; 2015 [Available from: http://www.un.org/sustainabledevelopment/.
2. Ackland M, Choi BCK, Puska P. Rethinking the terms non-communicable disease and chronic disease. British Medical Journal 2003;57(11):838-9.
3. Merriam-Webster. Merriam-Webster's Medical Dictionary Accessed 2006 26th October. Merriam-Webster Incorporated, 2002.
4. WHO. Global Strategy on Diet, Physical Activity and Health. Geneva: World Health Organisation, 2004.
5. Geleijnse JM, Kok FJ, Grobbee DE. Impact of dietary and lifestyle factors in the prevalence of hypertension in Western populations. European Journal of Public Health. 2004;14(3):235-9.
6. Cannon G (ed). Food, Nutrition and the Prevention of Cancer: a global perspective. Washington DC: World Cancer Research Fund / American Institute for Cancer Research; 1997.
7. Olivier S. Eat Your Heart Out. Nursing Standard. 2000;15(9):20-3.
8. Ashwell M. Concepts of Functional Foods. Brussels: International Life Sciences Institute Europe, 2002.
9. WHO. Diet, Nutrition and the Prevention of Chronic Diseases: Report of a Joint WHO/FAO Expert Consultation. Geneva: World Health Organisation, 2003.
10. Ettinger S. Macronutrients: Carbohydrates, Proteins and Lipids. In: Mahan LK, Escott-Stump S (eds). Krause's Food, Nutrition & Diet Therapy. 11th ed. Philadelphia: Saunders - Elsevier, 2004.
11. Gallagher ML. Vitamins. In: Mahan LK, Escott-Stump S (eds). Krause's Food, Nutrition & Diet Therapy. 11th ed. Philadelphia: Saunders-Elsevier, 2004.
12. Anderson JJB. Minerals. In: Mahan LK, Escott-Stump S (eds). Krause's Food, Nutrition & Diet Therapy. 11th ed. Philadelphia: Saunders-Elsevier, 2004.

13. Beyer P. Digestion, Absorption, Transport and Excretion of Nutrients. In: Mahan LK, Escott-Stump S (eds). Krause's Nutrition, Diet & Food Therapy. 11th ed. Philadelphia: Saunders-Elsevier, 2004.
14. Murray MT, Bongiorno PB. Role of Dietary Fibre in Health and Disease. In: Pizzorno JE, Murray MT (eds). Textbook of Natural Medicine. 3rd ed. Volume 1. St Louis: Churchill Livingstone Elsevier, 2006.
15. Jensen MK, Koh-Bannergee P, Hu FB, et al. Intakes of whole grains, bran, and germ and the risk of coronary heart disease in men. The American Journal of Clinical Nutrition. 2004(80):1492-9.
16. Tortora GJ, Derrickson B. Principles of Anatomy and Physiology. 11 ed. Hoboken: John Wiley & Sons Inc.; 2006.
17. Nowak TJ, Handford AG. Pathophysiology: Concepts and Applications for Health Care Professionals. 3rd ed. New York: McGraw - Hill Companies Ltd; 2004.
18. WHO. World Health Organisation Report 2004 - Changing History. Geneva: World Health Organisation, 2004.
19. Thiel RJ. Naturopathy For The 21st Century. Warsaw: Wendell W Whitman Company; 2000.

LEARNING SESSION TWO: CARBOHYDRATES AND LIPIDS, WHAT THEY ARE AND WHAT THEY DO

Introduction

We will follow on here from the very brief introduction that we had to carbohydrates in the previous learning session. What we know so far is that carbohydrates are essentially derived from plants and that 'triose's' (simple three carbon molecules) are the basic building blocks of sugars that form starches. We also know that lipids are the building blocks of fats and are found in both animal and plant-derived foods. There are three types of lipids; the essential fatty acids, triglycerides and phospholipids. Now we move on to the structure of carbohydrates and fats, what they are made up of and how they are structured. We go on to show how this relates to their function in the human body.

Following this basic explanation, we focus on carbohydrates and their role as a major supplier of energy. We look at the foods that supply us with carbohydrates and which ones give us the most nutrients for the energy content and which give the least. We look at the good carbohydrates and those that might be less than beneficial. In the final sections, we look again at fats and the necessity for essential fatty acids. We look at the right kinds of fats and the wrong kind and which fat-rich foods benefit us the most.

We then move on to the learning together sessions where we will engage in two activities in groups, which should provide a little light relief as well as helping to consolidate what everyone has learned so far. Help, as in the previous session, will be on hand from your facilitator. Finally, we come to the general discussion and the controversial subjects of dieting and the low carbohydrate and low-fat diets that have recently become popular.

What Carbohydrates and Fats are Composed of, the Similarities and Differences in Structure and Function

Carbohydrates

Both carbohydrates and lipids are composed of molecules of carbon, hydrogen and oxygen. Plants pick up carbon dioxide (CO_2) from the air and water (H_2O) from the soil and combine these to form carbohydrates in the process we know as photosynthesis. This is achieved by using both sunlight and chlorophyll enzymes to bring about a chemical reaction. Carbohydrate is a chemical name for hydrate (water) of carbon. This name is derived from the early investigations of scientists, who found that heating sugars for a long period of time, produced droplets of water, and a black residue which they identified as carbon which they release along with carbon dioxide, heat and energy. This process happens in the body as well during the metabolism of carbohydrates (used to produce energy)[1]. Although plants have the ability to pick up carbon dioxide from the air and water from the ground animals, do not, hence all of their carbohydrate has to be eaten in the form of plants (or from the intestines of animals that they kill for food)[1].

Carbohydrates are separated into two categories, simple and complex. Simple carbohydrates are in the form of sugars. Complex carbohydrates are in the form of long chains of hundreds or thousands of sugars and are commonly referred to as starches.

$$
\begin{array}{c}
CH{=}O \\
| \\
H{-}C{-}OH \\
| \\
HO{-}C{-}H \\
| \\
H{-}C{-}OH \\
| \\
H{-}C{-}OH \\
| \\
CH_2{-}OH
\end{array}
\qquad C_6H_{12}O_6
$$

(Would you like to count them up?)

Glucose [2]

This is the basic structure of glucose which is the simplest sugar molecule. A glucose molecule plus a fructose molecule together make sucrose, the simple sugar we know in crystalline form as table sugar. Many glucose molecules linked together form chains of molecules to become starch which is harder to break down and takes longer to digest. The structure of plant carbohydrates accounts for their variation in physiological properties, including their degree of sweetness and the rate of digestion and absorption [3].

The structure of the carbohydrate molecule is linked to its function. As a general rule, the simpler the carbohydrate molecule, the sweeter the substance and the more easily and quickly it is broken down by the body and absorbed [3]. Glucose is oxidised in the body to give energy and heat:

$$C_6H_{12}O_6 + 6O_2 \rightarrow \qquad 6CO_2 + \qquad\qquad 6H_2O + Energy + Heat$$

Glucose   Carbon Dioxide   Water

Complex carbohydrates in the form of both digestible and non-digestible starches are broken down more slowly maintaining a steady flow of glucose and energy. The non-digestible portion of the carbohydrate slows down the absorption and provides a fermentable base for the production of health-enhancing 'friendly' bacteria in the large intestines [3]. Carbohydrates can be classified as:

- Monosaccharides (single sugars) such as glucose and fructose
- Disaccharides (double sugars) and oligosaccharides (a few sugars) such as sucrose, lactose and maltose
- Polysaccharides (many sugars) such as starches and non-digestible polymers (fibres, pectins and gums)

Glucose is the most widely distributed sugar in nature although it is usually consumed in the form of starches and cellulose. Glucose linked with fructose to form sucrose makes up a large fraction of the content of fruits and vegetables, alongside some of the non-digestible starches. Fructose is the sweetest of all the monosaccharides, and between 1% and 7% fructose can be found in most fruits. As the fruit ripens, enzymes split the sucrose molecules into glucose and fructose which results in a sweeter taste. Fructose makes up about 3% of vegetables and 40% of honey. Galactose is another simple sugar but hardly found in nature except for breast milk, together with glucose it forms the basis of lactose, the disaccharide found in dairy products, especially milk [3].

Disaccharides are formed from two glucose molecules, or glucose and a fructose molecule by a glycosidic linkage between the OH groups in the molecules (you really don't have to remember this, it is just for interest!). Once this glycosidic bond is formed the position is 'frozen'. Random linkages between hydroxyl (OH) groups create a wide variety of disaccharides and oligosaccharides. The most common form of disaccharide is sucrose – known commonly in its crystalline form as table sugar and, in its natural form, it is found in sugar cane and beets [3]. Lactose is commonly known as 'milk sugar' and comprises 4.5% of cow's milk. Disaccharides are not quite as sweet as monosaccharides and, are not directly absorbed by the body the link between them needs to be broken down first to split them into monosaccharides. This requires the enzymes invertase (to split sucrose), maltase (to split maltose) and lactase (to split lactose). The insufficiency of the latter is sometimes a problem which occurs predominantly in those of Asian and African origin and about 10% of Europeans[3].

Plants store carbohydrates as starch by linking chains of glucose into a complex granular structure. The more carbohydrate the plant makes during photosynthesis, the greater the rate of starch formation. Edible plants make two types of starch; amylase which is a smaller, less complex structure and amylopectin, which has a very high molecular weight. Amylopectin is more abundant in the food supply and makes up a greater portion of the starch in tubers such as potatoes, sweet potatoes and yams and in grains such as corn, rice and oats. Starches are found mainly in grains, roots, tubers and plantains as well as pulses, (which also contain a significant amount of protein)[4]. Because the structure is complex, raw starch cannot be broken down and requires moist cooking which causes the cells containing the starch molecules to swell and gelatinise, rupturing the cell walls and making it more digestible. Some starch remains (resistant starch) yielding limited amounts of glucose for absorption. Starch releases glucose slowly and is therefore useful in sustaining energy over a longer period of time[3].

Fats

Lipid is the chemical name for a group of compounds which includes fats, oils and fat-related substances such as cholesterol and lecithin. Fats and lipids too, have a simple structure of carbon, hydrogen and oxygen atoms and, like carbohydrates, their properties and functions in the body are also linked closely to their structure. Lipids are compounds that frequently occur in nature and are an important part of the plant, animal and microbial membranes. The definition of a lipid is based on its solubility. Whilst carbohydrates are soluble in water, lipids are only marginally soluble in water (at best) and are soluble in organic solvents such as acetone and chloroform. Fats and oils are typical lipids in terms of their solubility [5].

Lipids may be simple or compound, and both yield fatty acids, which are straight-chain organic acids. The fatty acids that are found in nature all contain an even number of carbon atoms [1]. A lipid is referred to as fat if it is solid at room temperature and oil if it is liquid at room temperature. Lipids from animal sources are usually solid and therefore fats, and those from vegetable sources are usually liquid and are therefore oils. Lipids constitute just over a third (34%) of the energy intake of the average diet and can store energy in the form of fats in adipocytes, the cells that form adipose tissue. The ability to store and use large amounts of fats originally enabled humans to survive without food for weeks, or even months, during periods of drought, cold and famine. This ability contributed to the survival of early humans [3].

The three types of lipids that we are most concerned with in nutrition are the fatty acids, the triglycerides and the phospholipids. The fatty acids are those that we need to be most aware of as it is these that are essential as far as our food intake is concerned [3].

The basic formula for fats is: $C_{12}H_{24}O_2$

Different types of fatty acids have different lengths of carbon chains, meaning that the number of carbon atoms and hydrogen atoms increases in proportion to one another depending on the fatty acid[5].

$$H_3C \diagup \overset{CH_2}{\underset{CH_2}{\diagup}} \overset{CH_2}{\underset{CH_2}{\diagup}} \overset{CH_2}{\underset{CH_2}{\diagup}} \overset{CH_2}{\underset{CH_2}{\diagup}} \overset{CH_2}{\diagup} CH_2 \text{---} COOH$$

Lauric Acid [2]

Above is a simple fatty acid chain showing the carbon, hydrogen and oxygen atoms.

In addition, there are both saturated and unsaturated fatty acids – this relates to the way in which the atoms are bonded together [5]. If all the available bonds are used up (i.e. there is no extra space for another atom or molecule to attach itself), then the fat is said to be 'saturated'. Saturated fat will always have twice the number of hydrogen atoms as carbon atoms, one per bond. If there are, however, some double bonds between the carbon and hydrogen atoms, then the fat is said to be unsaturated. This essentially means that it has 'space for another atom of hydrogen or to connect to another molecule' which is important when we look at how fats are hardened by adding hydrogen to them, or how they combine with phosphorous to make phospholipids, or proteins to make hormones. A monounsaturated fatty acid has a single, double bond, and polyunsaturated fatty acids have two or more double bonds [5].

The three essential fatty acids all have double bonds and are unsaturated. Linoleic acid is nutritionally the most essential as it cannot be synthesised by the human body however linolenic acid can be synthesised from it. Linoleic acid is found mainly in linseed oil and also in corn, peanut and soybean oils [3].

- Oleic Acid $C_{18}H_{34}O_2$ 1 double bond
- Linoleic Acid $C_{18}H_{32}O_2$ 2 double bonds
- Alpha Linolenic Acid $C_{18}H_{30}O_2$ 3 double bonds

There are some differences between saturated and unsaturated fatty acids that are linked to their respective structures. The structure, in turn, is related to the function of the fats, in the case of saturated fats the main purpose is to provide a source of stored energy in the adipocytes. Because saturated fatty acids contain more hydrogen and have no double bonds, they have certain properties:

- They are mainly solid at room temperature
- They are relatively stable
- They are found predominantly in animal fat

Unsaturated fatty acids, however, have different properties and serve different functions in the body mainly, that of providing a flexible lipid membrane for the body's cells:

- They are fluid at room temperature
- They possess a degree of instability, especially when heated
- They are found predominantly in vegetable oils, nuts, seeds and, to a lesser extent, in cold water fish

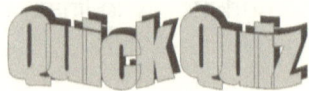

True or False?

1. Both carbohydrates and lipids are composed of molecules containing the elements carbon, hydrogen and nitrogen

    _____

2. Photosynthesis is achieved by using sunlight and chlorophyll enzymes to bring about a chemical reaction in plants

    _____

3. The formula for glucose is $C_{12}H_{24}O_2$

    _____

4. The body breaks down complex carbohydrates very quickly but simple carbohydrates more slowly

    _____

5. The basic formula for lipids is $C_6H_{12}O_6$

    _____

6. The most nutritionally essential lipids are the fatty acids

    _____

7. Fatty acids all have the same length carbon chain

    _____

8. An unsaturated fatty acid has more single bonds than a saturated fatty acid

    _____

9. Saturated fatty acids are more stable, especially when heated

    _____

10. Salad and cooking oil would contain predominantly unsaturated fatty acids

    _____

The Role of Carbohydrates in Providing Energy

Carbohydrates are the main source of energy in most countries in the world and the metabolically 'preferred' source of energy for the body. Carbohydrates are made up of starches, non-starch polysaccharides (NSP, the major component of dietary fibre), which are usually termed complex carbohydrates, as well as monosaccharides and disaccharides, usually termed simple sugars. These are chemically very similar but vary in their physiological effects. In most parts of the developing world 50-80% of the total energy taken in comes from carbohydrate-rich foods, a proportion of carbohydrate that has kept the human race from extinction and allowed it to grow and flourish for many thousands of years. However, with economic development, the proportion of energy taken in from carbohydrate foods drops to 40-50% of the total energy intake, of which an increasing amount comes from refined simple sugars. As less unrefined and complex starch is consumed the amount of NSP in the diet also decreases [4].

A growing body of evidence now suggests that dietary carbohydrates, especially NSP, have a significant impact on the human physiology. Specific carbohydrates modulate whole-body energy processes and, in addition, affect certain disease processes. Carbohydrates in all forms are broken down by enzymes which split the glycosidic links holding the molecules of monosaccharides together. The ability to digest carbohydrate is modified by three factors [3]:

- The relative availability of the type of carbohydrate to the action of digestive enzymes
- The level of activity of the digestive enzymes – this is particularly important in the case of lactase as some people do not have adequate levels of this enzyme
- The presence of factors such as dietary fats and dietary fibre, both of which slow the stomach emptying and the rate of digestion of carbohydrates

The fewer the glycosidic linkages, the quicker the process, which is why monosaccharides, which do not require enzymatic action, and disaccharides with only one link to break down are absorbed from the digestive system and enter the bloodstream very quickly. This is especially the case in the absence of dietary fibre. More complex carbohydrates, however, require a longer chemical process of splitting the numerous glycosidic links, releasing the individual molecules much more slowly into the system. In addition, unrefined complex carbohydrates are more likely to be bound together with significant amounts of NSP and some small amounts of dietary fats, thus allowing for a longer, slower process of digestion and absorption [3].

The net result of such a process is that simple carbohydrates and foods containing predominantly monosaccharides and disaccharides are broken down and released into the bloodstream in a short amount of time. This elevates the blood glucose levels which in turn, triggers the pancreas into releasing insulin. Insulin is a hormone that carries the glucose molecule across the cell wall, thus providing some of the 'starter material' for the production of energy within the body's cells [3]. We will return again to the issue of control of blood glucose levels and what happens at the cellular level later in session nine.

The brain is the most important recipient of glucose from the blood, without a steady and constant stream of glucose crossing the blood-brain barrier the brain cannot function adequately[6]. Periodic surges in blood glucose trigger insulin release which carries the glucose into the cells, however, with constant 'priming' for insulin release the pancreas can become oversensitive, releasing too much insulin too quickly, resulting in dips in the level of glucose below the amount necessary for optimum brain function. This accounts for a problem known as food stimulated or 'reactive' hypoglycaemia, the symptoms of which include sudden hunger, cravings for sweets, anxiety, shakiness, cold sweats, pallor and disorientation or confusion[7].

The glycaemic index is used to rank different dietary carbohydrates on their ability to raise blood glucose levels. It basically gives an indication of how long it takes to split the glycosidic links in a particular food, digest it completely and absorb the glucose into the bloodstream. The higher the food on the index (ranking close to 100), the quicker it reaches the bloodstream. Foods that are lower on the index (below 60) are slower burning, but eventually, all of the food is broken down and absorbed albeit, at a much more steady and reliable pace. The benefit of such foods is that when one consumes these, one feels more satisfied and sustains a steady energy level for longer[3]. Use of the glycaemic index for self-monitoring of diets for people with diabetes and other dietary related problems is under investigation, as it could be a useful way of controlling the levels of blood glucose. It has also been used, however, in some popular weight loss diets, including high protein and high-fat type diets and those that simply restrict carbohydrate to a certain level. While such diets have been used successfully in weight reduction in the short term there is little research to suggest that the weight loss would be sustained over the longer term[8]. To be taken into consideration is that such diets that are particularly low in carbohydrates have been known to cause complications from the restriction of certain fruits, vegetables, and grains that contain essential vitamins and minerals, as well as the restriction in dietary fibre which has the potential to generate problems in the lower intestines in the longer term [4]. An indication of the glycaemic index of some foods in general use:

Food	GI	Food	GI
Glucose	100	Baked Beans	48
Cornflakes	92	Orange	48
Potato – boiled	88	Carrots	47
White rice	87	Grapes	46
Cocoa puffs	77	Apple	38
Whole wheat bread	77	Yam	37
Pumpkin	75	Butter beans	31
White bread	70	All bran	30
Rye crispbread	69	Lentils	29

Special K	69	Chickpeas	28
Sucrose (table sugar)	68	Kidney beans	28
Canned beetroot	64	Milk	27
Sweet-corn	60	Grapefruit	25
Whole grain rye bread	58	Cherries	22
Pita bread	57	Soybeans	18
Oat crackers	55	Peanuts	14
Banana	51	Green vegetables, salads and	
Brown Rice	50	most fish rank below this level	

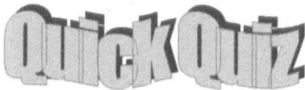

True or False?

1. Non-Starch Polysaccharides are the major components ofsimple sugars

   _____

2. In developed Westernised countries 50-80% of the diet consists of carbohydrates

   _____

3. The ability to digest carbohydrates can depend on the activity of digestive enzymes

   _____

4. Dietary fats slow down the digestion and absorption of carbohydrates

   _____

5. In the absence of dietary fibre, carbohydrates are broken down more quickly

   _____

6. The liver is the most important recipient of glucose from the blood

   _____

7. The pancreas can become oversensitive when the body experiences too many sudden surges in blood glucose levels

   _____

8. One can restrict carbohydrates without any complications in order to lose weight

   _____

9. The glycaemic index tells us how much or how little carbohydrate we absorb from food

   _____

10. The glycaemic index tells us how quickly the carbohydrate in a given food is broken down and absorbed

   _____

Carbohydrate-Rich Foods: Good, Better, Better Still!

When taking into consideration how much carbohydrate to take in and what type of carbohydrate it is best to eat, we need to take in other factors besides the speed at which carbohydrate metabolises and turns into blood glucose. These include:

- The NSP, or fibre content of the food
- The degree of processing the food has undergone
- The micronutrient density (MD) of the food

The trick with carbohydrate consumption is not to restrict carbohydrates *per se* as this can lead to many other problems, including those resulting from lack of fibre and insufficient anti-oxidant nutrients (we will come to these in learning sessions 4, 5 and 6). There is a good amount of evidence to support the value of eating plenty of carbohydrates in the form of fresh fruits and vegetables, whole grain pasta and pulses to reduce our risk of diseases such as cancer [4], hypertension and stroke, [9] cardiac heart disease [10] and the problems inherent in ageing,[11] including macular degeneration which is a leading cause of blindness in older people [12].

Unrefined carbohydrate-rich foods have enormous benefits if we choose them wisely, including:

- Regulating blood glucose levels and providing a steady, stable stream of energy to the body's cells including those in the brain
- Providing adequate amounts of dietary fibre which regulates fat absorption and controls the amount of undesirable fats absorbed into the bloodstream
- Providing most of our water-soluble and many of our fat-soluble vitamins
- Providing our best sources of many essential minerals

The effects of refining carbohydrates, however, remove much of the fibre and many of the B-complex vitamins and minerals. This has the effect of speeding up the time it takes to break the glycosidic links and facilitate absorption as well as lowering the nutritional content of the food item overall.

The NSP content of food of vegetable or plant origin is often directly related to the amount of refinement it has undergone. Highly refined foods have much of the cellulose and hemicellulose removed as well as the pips, kernels, or seeds that contain lignins and gums. NSP not only aids in moving the food through the gastrointestinal tract at an appropriate pace but have other functions too, including the regulation of fat absorption, as well as playing a major role in the immune function.

The micronutrient density (MD) of the diet is something we will discuss in depth later in the course; however, essentially the micronutrient density is the ratio of micronutrients to potential energy a food contains. Foods which are high in potential energy, or calorific value, but have few micronutrients due to processing and cooking practices are low nutrient micronutrient density (low MD), and those that have a high micronutrient value and fewer calories have a high MD.

When we are making decisions about carbohydrate consumption we need to look at the following:

- The glycaemic index (GI)
- The amount of refining the food has undergone
- The fibre content of the food
- The micronutrient density (MD)
- Whether or not it is culturally acceptable

The last point is quite important as, when making decisions about diet and food intake over the longer term, we will not stick to something that is not culturally acceptable no matter how much we might wish to. This is very important when we are planning meals for our families and others we care for. Some things are, however, a matter of acquired taste and habit, which can be changed over a period of time.

Good sources of carbohydrate have a moderate GI of between 55 and 75, are relatively unrefined and have a moderate amount of fibre and micronutrient content. Better sources have a glycaemic index of less than 55, are less refined and have a higher fibre content and micronutrient density, or they have a high GI index score but are totally unrefined and have a high MD. Best sources combine the benefits of unrefined foods with a GI below 50, a high NSP content and high MD.

A few examples are given below:

GOOD

Shredded wheat	Rye crisp breads	Winter squash
Weetabix	Whole wheat crackers	Turnips
Sorghum	Baked Potatoes	Popcorn
Oatcakes	New Potatoes	Split pea soup
Basmati Rice	Sweet Potato	Paw Paw
Wholegrain pasta	Sweet Corn	Watermelon
Granary breads	Beetroot	Raisins
Wholegrain Rye Bread	Rutabaga	Cantaloupe
Brown Pita Bread	Pumpkin	Pineapple

BETTER

Whole wheat bread	Artichokes – globe	Dates
Millet	Artichokes – Jerusalem	Figs
Oats porridge	Wax Beans	Grapes
Buckwheat	Carrots	
Muesli – home made	Fresh peas	
Wholegrain brown rice	Onions	

BETTER STILL

Yams	Pears	Green vegetables
Bananas and Plantains	All Berries	Salad vegetables
Kiwi Fruit	Apricots	Mushrooms

Oranges	Peaches	Summer squash
Apples	Plums	Snow peas
All citrus fruit	Tomatoes	*All pulses

* These are also a good source of vegetable protein

The above list is not exhaustive and no doubt you can find some examples from your own cultural foods. Some foods in the 'best category' are there because of their low glycaemic index and high micronutrient density, but they are not very filling, so meals need to be made from a combination of these foods to reach an overall moderate GI level and a reasonable level of micronutrients and fibre. We will do this together later in the programme when we look at meal planning.

Some of the less satisfactory sources of carbohydrates include those that are highly processed, or refined and, of a high GI and low MD. Such food includes white bread, processed sweetened breakfast cereals, pastries and cakes, sugar, jams and confectionary and many dessert items. Whilst these do contain carbohydrate that breaks down into glucose they do not contain much else and are not good 'nutritional value'.

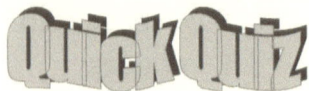

True or False?

1. Good sources of carbohydrate combine low glycaemic index with high fibre and micronutrient content

   _____

2. How processed or refined a source of carbohydrate is, is not as important as how much starch it contains

   _____

3. The best sources of carbohydrate are the ones that are the least refined and have the highest micronutrient density

   _____

4. White bread and jam would be a good source of carbohydrate because it combines a quickly broken-down food with a more slowly broken down food

   _____

The Necessity for Lipids and Fats

Lipids have many vital functions in the body. They account for 15% of the normal body weight of men and 20% of the normal body weight of women. At least half of this is stored under the skin as adipose tissue, the rest provides insulation, cushions vital organs, and carries nutrients in the blood. Adipose tissue is made of fat storage cells where most fat under the skin is stored. This fat can be burned for energy provided carbohydrate is present. Fat as an energy source is very concentrated providing nine calories per gram as against carbohydrate and protein which provide four calories per gram. Lipids are present in cell membranes and transport vitamins A, D, E, and K through the body. Lipids are carriers of essential fatty acids; polyunsaturated fats provide linoleic acid. Deficiency of this causes red and scaly skin, stunted growth in children, dehydration and infections.

Lipids increase the palatability of foods by enhancing their taste, flavour, juiciness and tenderness. Dietary fat has several essential functions related to digestion and absorption as well as utilisation of other nutrients. Primarily dietary fat as discussed earlier gives one a feeling of satiety and prevents overeating to some extent. It also delays gastric emptying time which allows the digestive enzymes to work and stimulates the flow of pancreatic juices and bile (two important components of digestive juices). In summary, fats are essential for:

- Transport of fat-soluble vitamins
- Production of steroids and hormones in the body
- The integrity of individual cell membranes

Like carbohydrates, lipids may be simple or compound. Simple lipids include the fatty acids and neutral fats. These are fatty acids bound to glycerol and include triglycerides. Compound lipids are fatty acids bound to phosphoric acid and another nitrogen-based molecule (generally a protein), such as the phospholipids and lipoproteins [3]. We have discussed what the essential fatty acids are and mentioned that phospholipids and triglycerides are also necessary to our health, but what exactly are the phospholipids and triglycerides and what do they do?

Triglycerides

Fatty acids are rarely found 'free' in nature as they are dangerous due to the potential reactivity of the carboxylic part (COOH) of the molecule, which can react with other molecules resulting in tissue damage. Biologic organisms, therefore, link three fatty acids to a molecule of glycerol to form a triglyceride. Most lipids in foods (more than 95%) and also in the body are in the form of triglycerides. When we are talking about fat, either in food or in the body, we really are talking about triglycerides. Fatty acids linked to glycerol are usually neutral, they can be safely transported in the blood and stored in fat cells (adipose tissue) without doing any damage [3].

Although bound together with glycerol to form triglycerides, fatty acids and therefore triglycerides retain the length of their chains and degree of saturation and thus their natural properties. The triglycerides in foods reflect the needs of the organism from where they have come. Thus, storage triglycerides from animal products are mainly saturated; however, cold-water creatures must maintain their triglycerides in liquid form even at low temperatures. Therefore the triglycerides in fish oils and marine fats are highly unsaturated [3].

Phospholipids

Phospholipids are triglycerides that contain a phosphate molecule, attached to the triglyceride at one end and at the other end to a nitrogen-containing molecule (usually choline, serine or inositol). The phosphate-containing portion of this molecule forms hydrogen bonds with water, thus making the whole phospholipid more soluble in water and giving it the ability to carry the fat portions into the digestive juices, thus enabling the digestion and absorption of fats[3].

A very important phospholipid is phosphatidylcholine (commonly known as lecithin), which is used to transport fats and cholesterol in the body. Lecithin is so essential to the body, as it is a component of cell membranes and has been found in the memory cells of the brain, that it can be manufactured in the liver. Lecithin acts as a fat emulsifier, keeping it in solution in the blood and in other parts of the body. Lecithin is widely distributed in the food chain, the best sources being egg yolks, soybeans, peanuts, legumes and spinach [3].

Cholesterol

Cholesterol is probably the best-known fat related compound. It belongs to a class of lipid substances called sterols. It is obtained from certain foods those containing saturated and animal fats; however, the body also manufactures cholesterol from adipose fat, sugars, and amino acids 'going spare', consumed in excess, or not needed by the body's cells.

Cholesterol is widely distributed in our body's cells and is a vital component of the cell membrane. It is also found in large amounts of the brain and nerve tissue, and it forms the steroid base of all the sex hormones. A cholesterol derivative which lies under the surface of the skin cells reacts to sunlight on the skin and forms vitamin D, which carries bone-building minerals from the blood to the bone cells. Cholesterol is also used in making bile acids that function in the digestion of fats. Cholesterol in food is found in organ meats, eggs, dairy products, meat, poultry, fish and shellfish.

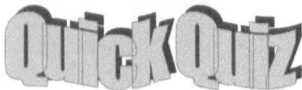

True or False?

1. Phospholipids are essential and cannot be manufactured in the body   _____

2. Triglycerides consist of two fatty acids and a glycerol molecule   _____

3. Fatty acids are rarely found free in nature   _____

4. Fatty acids are characterised by the number of double bonds   _____

The Right Kinds of Fats and the Wrong Kind of Fats

Fat is the most energy dense constituent of the diet, and its contribution to dietary energy rises with industrialisation and urbanisation of the population. Oils and fats are present in most foods to a greater or lesser extent; however, meat from domesticated animals has a high-fat content as have many manufactured foods, in addition, oils and fats are often added at the table[4]. Also, food often contains a mixture of both saturated and unsaturated triglycerides and phospholipids, which bind to a greater or lesser degree with proteins. In this form, we refer to them as lipoproteins. It is in the form of lipoproteins that fats are carried around in the blood. High-density lipoproteins (HDL) contain more proteins and fewer triglycerides and cholesterol and aid in clearing the less good fats from the system. Low-density lipoproteins (LDL) arise out of saturated fats and trans-fatty acids from processed foods and, carry the greater portion of cholesterol in the blood. LDLs also are responsible for the damage to the lining of the blood vessels [13]. In the fight against cardiac disease and cancer, it has been found to be overall beneficial to have more HDL than LDL in the blood [4,13].

Some fats are useful, some are less useful, and some are not useful at all. In this section, we will explore what kinds of fats are most useful and where and how to obtain them from the food sources available to us. In order to make decisions about fat consumption, we need to take several things into consideration with respect to the construction of the lipids in the foods we are consuming[4,13].

- The degree of saturation
- The position of the double bonds in unsaturated fats
- The ideal ratio of fats for health and well-being

The Degree of Saturation

The degree of saturation is important as all of the essential fatty acids are unsaturated, the saturated ones are those that are not essential and, in some instances, can do some harm. Generally, saturated fats are best avoided, or at least limited. These are found mainly in [3,4]:

- Butter, cheeses and full-fat dairy products
- Red meats, pork, most game meats
- Chicken, turkey and duck
- Shellfish and seafood
- Processed items such as spreads, pates and many baked goods
- Coconut and palm oils

There are, however, some foods which, although they contain saturated fats, do so in smaller amounts and have other additional nutritional benefits:

- Eggs – these are highly nutritious and are a good source of Vitamin B12, iron, Vitamin A and, in addition, contain lecithin which helps to emulsify the cholesterol content. Eggs are an excellent source of protein.
- Yoghurt – good quality low-fat probiotic yoghurt has the benefits of containing 'friendly' bacteria that aid the digestive system and the immune system.
- Fish – contains generally less fat, a greater portion of which is unsaturated and beneficial.

Monosaturated fatty acids have one double bond, the best example being olive oil; however, the cooked olives preserved either in water or olive oil are even better, as they contain more micronutrients. Olive oil does not deteriorate or change its structure when heated to a moderate degree, so it is a relatively safe oil to cook with. Canola oil also has only one double bond and is, therefore, monosaturated it is often a good choice for salad dressing if one wishes to avoid the very strong taste of olive oil.

Polyunsaturated fats are those with more than one double bond, in foods, this is usually two or three double bonds. These are more beneficial to health and are the precursors of 'good' HDL in the bloodstream. Food sources include [3]:

- Nuts, and seeds
- Avocado pears
- Legumes (Soybeans and peanuts)
- Grain oils (corn, wheat germ) and whole grains
- Cold water fish

The Position of The Double Bonds

Fatty acids are characterised by the position or location of the double bonds within the molecule. The most common convention of describing where these are is to count the double bonds from the last carbon in the fatty acid chain, then precede that number by the Greek symbol ώ, (omega), this being the fatty acid's omega number. Double bonds are counted from the last carbon in the chain. Linoleic acid has 18 carbons and 2 double bonds the first of which is six carbons from the end making it an ώ6 fatty acid. Alpha-linolenic acid has 18 carbons and 3 double bonds, the first of which is 3 carbons from the end, giving it the designation of ώ3 fatty acid. Cold water fish oils are composed of eicosapentaenoic acid (EPA) which has 20 carbons and five double bonds, the first being three carbons from the end making it a polyunsaturated ώ3 fatty acid. Oleic acid (from olives, olive and canola oils) has 18 carbons and one double bond which is 9 carbons from the end and is designated an ώ9 fatty acid. Since the essential fatty acids are predominantly omega 3, 6 or 9 fatty acids, it is these that we are concerned with [3].

The Ideal Ratio of Fats

It has been postulated that humans evolved by consuming a diet lower in saturated fat and higher in ώ3 fatty acids than is consumed today. Ancient peoples either lived by the oceans and consumed fish and fruits or lived inland and consumed a diet far higher in plant foods, high in ώ3 than currently consumed [14]. The Palaeolithic diet is thought to have been richer in marine and plant sources of ώ3 fats and lower in ώ6 fats resulting in a ratio of 1:1 ώ3: ώ6. In contrast, the modern diet is richer in ώ6 from both animal protein and oils extracted from grains such as corn and safflower oils [3]. To date there is a variation in what has been considered an optimal ratio; at present, it is recommended that the ώ6: ώ3 ratio should be between 2:1 and 3:1 which is approximately four times lower than the current average intake of ώ6 fatty acids [3]. Also, ώ9 fats, as in olive oil, are to be taken into consideration as some benefit has been shown from a diet which features olive oil as opposed to more saturated oils or refined grain extracted oils [10,15]. Perhaps considering the research available a prudent ratio of fats might be: **3ώ6: 2ώ3: 1ώ9**.

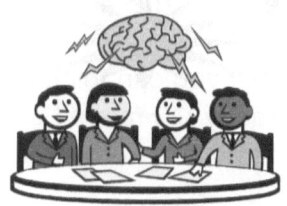

Learning Together

Learning Together

Activity 2.1: Allow yourselves 15 minutes for this activity

From what you now know about carbohydrates:

What do you think is the difference between whole-grain brown rice and refined white rice?

Do you think that 2- 3 hours after eating a meal based on whole grain brown rice you would be more or less hungry than if you had the same meal with white rice?

Why do you think this is so?

Write Your Notes Here

Activity 2.2: Allow yourselves 10 minutes for this activity

From the information, you have been given see if you can think up a meal that you could eat that had twice as many ẇ3 fats as ẇ6 fats and as little saturated fat as possible. Write down the menu / ingredients for the meal below.

Write Your Notes Here

Now you should take 5 minutes to discuss the answers with your facilitator

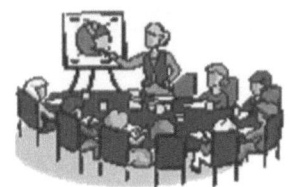

Discussion

Today's Topic for Discussion is: 'LOW CARBOHYDRATE AND LOW-FAT DIETING'

A group of researchers looked at four very popular weight loss diets [8]:

- South Beach: a three-phase diet which starts off severely restricting carbohydrate and then gradually phases some of it back in, ending with a low GI diet as a maintenance plan
- Sugar Busters! a two-week plan that cuts out sugar and refined sugary foods rather than carbohydrate, the diet emphasises GI and advocates against overdoing any type of carbohydrate foods long term.
- Ornish: Dietary fat is restricted severely to 10% of total calories and includes 70% of calories from complex high fibre carbohydrates with a restriction on sugars
- EatRight: This is a 12-week lifestyle plan that restricts the calorie intake and emphasises large quantities of high fibre low-calorie foods in the form of fruits, vegetables and high fibre cereals with moderate amounts of meats, cheeses and sugar

In the final analysis, there was little difference between the South Beach, Sugar Busters and EatRight diets as the latter was calorie restricted and therefore restricted the overall carbohydrate intake. There is some suggestion of short-term weight loss on low carbohydrate diets [8]; however, the Ornish plan has been promoted as one that prevents cardiac heart disease [16]. Some questions to think about:

- As a group do you think that losing weight in the short term is more or less important than long-term nutritional balance?
- Do you think that any of the above programmes might result in nutritional or medical problems over the longer term?

<u>You Might Wish to Write Some Notes Here</u>

References

1. Sackheim GL, Lehman DD. Chemistry for the Health Sciences. 2nd ed. New York: Macmillan; 1994.
2. ACD. ACD/ChemSketch.v.10. Toronto ON: Advanced Chemistry Development Inc; 2006.
3. Ettinger S. Macronutrients: Carbohydrates, Proteins and Lipids. In: Mahan LK, Escott-Stump S (eds). Krause's Food Nutrition & Diet Therapy. 11th ed. Philadelphia: Saunders Elsevier, 2004.
4. Food, Nutrition and the Prevention of Cancer, a Global Perspective. Washington DC: World Cancer Research Fund / American Institute for Cancer Research, 1997.
5. Campbell MK. Biochemistry. 2nd ed. Orlando: Saunders; 1995.
6. Nowak TJ, Handford AG. Pathophysiology: Concepts and Applications for Health Care Professionals. 3rd ed. New York: The McGraw - Hill Companies Inc.; 2004.
7. Service FJ. Hypoglycaemias. Western Journal of Medicine. 1991;154:442-54.
8. Shikany JM, Thomas SE, Henson CS, Redden DT, Heimburger DC. Glycaemic Index and Glycaemic Load of Popular Weight-Loss Diets. Medscape General Medicine. Volume 1, 2006:22.
9. Brookes L. New Dietary Advice, a New Government Program, A New Drug and a Truly Novel New BP Measurement Device. Medscape Cardiology. Volume 10, 2006:523827.
10. Franco OH, Bonneaux L, deLaet C, Peeters A, Steyerberg EW, Machenbach JP. The Polymeal: a more natural, safer and probably tastier (than the polypill) strategy to reduce cardiovascular disease by more than 75%. British Medical Journal. 2004; 329:1447-50.
11. Frassetto L, Morris RC, Sellmeyer DE, Todd K, Sebastian A. Diet, evolution and ageing: The pathophysiological effects of the post-agricultural inversion of potassium-to-sodium and base-to-chloride ratios in the human diet. European Journal of Nutrition. 2001;40(5):200-13.

12. Barclay L, Lie D. High Dietary Antioxidant Intake May Reduce Risk for Age-Related Macular Degeneration. Medscape Medical News. 2006(520823).
13. Krummel DA. Medical Nutrition Therapy in Cardiovascular Disease. In: Mahan LK, Escott-Stump S (eds). Krause's Food, Nutrition & Diet Therapy. 11th ed. Philadelphia: Saunders Elsevier, 2004.
14. Crawford MA. The role of dietary fatty acids in biology; their place in the evolution of the human brain. Nutrition Reviews. 1992(50):3.
15. Trichopoulou A, Orfanos P, Norat T, et al. Modified Mediterranean diet and survival: EPIC-elderly prospective cohort study. British Medical Journal. Volume 10, 2005:1-7.
16. Ornish D. Eat More, Weigh Less: Dr Dean Ornish's Life choice Programme for Losing Weight Safely Whilst Eating Abundantly. New York: Quill; 2001.

LEARNING SESSION THREE: PROTEIN - WHAT IT IS AND THE SPECIAL ROLE IT HAS IN OUR HEALTH

Introduction

Remember Pvt. Tim Hall? Protein is the building block substance that ultimately determines whether there is life! Everything that lives, plants, trees, flowers, insects and animals and of course human beings are built on proteins. Other than water, proteins are the chief constituents of the human body. They make up the cells of tissues, especially muscle; epithelial tissue that forms the basis of skin, finger and toenails and hair; as well as the internal lining of the digestive system; the vascular system of arteries and veins; the respiratory system and all our organs. In addition, hormones, blood cells and other body chemicals also have a protein base, and the DNA and RNA that makes up the core master centre of the nucleus of our cells and our genetic characteristics are made up from the amino acids that form the building blocks of proteins.

There are 20 amino acids that human beings cannot live without, half of these can be manufactured in the body from a combination of the essential amino acids and other chemicals within our system. The other half are truly indispensable, and we can find ourselves in all sorts of trouble if we do not obtain them in our diet. To complicate matters further the amino acids are a little like a jigsaw puzzle, it is not just a case of numbers, but they have to 'fit' into a given pattern of 'completeness'.

This session will look at the amino acids and how they are constructed in nature, where we get them from in the food supply and how to get the amounts that we need to build our own bodily proteins without having too many of the ones that might, in excess, cause problems. We will discuss the quality vs quantity issue, combining protein and carbohydrate-rich foods and how to do this to our advantage without placing an overload on our digestive systems. We then move on to some 'fun stuff' and two learning together activities before discussing the question of how to obtain adequate protein and the question of meat eating vs. vegetarianism.

The Amino Acids and the Protein Molecules

Firstly, we have just a little bit of chemistry to explain the structure. Proteins are polymers; large molecules built up from smaller molecules called amino acids. Like carbohydrates and lipids, amino acids also contain carbon, hydrogen and oxygen; in addition, they contain nitrogen. The definition of an amino acid is an organic acid (COOH made up of carbon, oxygen and hydrogen) with an amine group (NH_2 – containing nitrogen) attached. The R group represents the attached atoms that form the rest of each of the particular amino acid molecules [1].

$$\begin{array}{c} COOH \\ | \\ H - C - NH_2 \\ | \\ R \end{array}$$

__A Basic Amino Acid Structure__ [2]

The nature of the attached R group will determine whether or not the particular amino acid is polar (soluble in water) or non-polar (not very soluble in water). Amino acids contain the COOH group which is acid as well as the NH_2 group which is basic (alkali) the whole molecule, therefore, is neutral; however, it may have the ability to react with either acids or bases to form more complex protein molecules [1].

$$\begin{array}{c} COOH \\ | \\ H - C - NH_2 \\ | \\ CH \\ \diagup \quad \diagdown \\ CH_3 \qquad HC_3 \end{array}$$

__Valine – (Non-Polar)__ [2]

$$COOH$$
$$|$$
$$H - C - NH_2 \longrightarrow$$

| Peptide Link |

$$|$$
$$OH - C - H$$
$$|$$
$$CH_3$$

Threonine – (Polar) [2]

The Essential and Non-Essential Amino Acids

The essential amino acids we have looked at before, in addition, there are another ten that our bodies make from the essential ones and that we need in order to function at our best – now we have the full picture [1]:

	Essential	Daily Requirement Mg/Kg			Non-Essential
		Adult	Infant		
P	Phenylalanine	22	135	G	Glutamine
V	Valine	35	93	A	Alanine
T	Threonine	28	87	S	Serine
				P	Proline
T	Tryptophan	33	12		
I	Isoleucine	28	70	C	Cysteine
M	Methionine	22	58	A	Asparginine
				T	Tyrosine
H	Histidine	-	28		
A	Arginine	-	-	G	Glycine
L	Lysine	44	103	A	Aspartic Acid
L	Leucine	42	161	G	Glutamic Acid

PVT TIM HALL took a GASP as the CAT told the GAG!

Essential amino acids can break down and re-form in order to make the non-essential ones, however, by having some of the non-essential amino acids in our foods we spare the essential ones, for the construction of proteins.

Proteins are polymers that are built up from many amino acids linked by a peptide bond (or peptide linkage). As molecules, they are much larger than either carbohydrates or lipids. Proteins contain many peptide bonds and the number of possible combinations of the many amino acids that form a given protein is beyond all comprehension, there are thousands, and we are still in the process of discovery!

Proteins are complex because they do so many 'jobs' in the human system, the molecules are very large, and this necessitates some form of arrangement whereby, despite their size and complexity, they take up as little space as possible. Nature has taken care of this in the way in which protein molecules are arranged. Initially, peptide bonds are formed between sequential amino acids, resulting in a linear chain known as the *primary structure* [3]. This primary structure refers to the number and sequence of the amino acids which are held together by peptide bonds, a slight change in the sequence can alter the entire protein and its function [1].

A straight chain of protein molecules
_____ **Primary Structure**

The *secondary structure* refers to the regularly recurring arrangement of the amino acid chain, which sometimes occurs as a pleated sheet, coil or a spiral [1]. This happens when attractions between the 'R' groups form new bonds resulting in the lines of molecules changing shape [3].

The chain of protein molecules either coils or bends like the one underneath

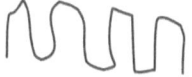

Secondary Structures

In more complex proteins the helixes and pleated sheets are folded into compact structures forming a *tertiary structure* [3] which folds the coils into layers or fibres, and it is this structure that given the particular protein their specific biological activity [1].

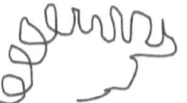

The coils or bends then coil in on themselves again

Tertiary Structure

Sometimes a protein will have a *quaternary structure* when different tertiary structure proteins combine to form an even more complex protein unit[1].

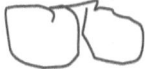

Quaternary Structure

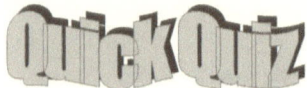

Using coloured pencils or pens place a circle around the words or labels given in the list below that you think are the ones being asked for:

1. Circle in red the essential amino acids

2. Circle in blue the non-essential amino acids

3. Circle in green the parts of the body constructed primarily out of proteins

4. Circle in orange the types of structure that proteins may have

5. How many amino acids do we require altogether? Circle the answer in yellow

Threonine   Methionine   Asparginine   Cysteine

Quaternary   Thousands   Valine   Tertiary

Fingernails   Ten   Simple   Phenylalanine   Glutamine

Twenty   Skin   Secondary   Complex

Adipose Tissue   Quadruple   Polysaccharide

Alanine   Hundreds   Muscles   Internal Organs

Millions   Body Fluids   Primary

The Functions of Protein and Its Importance in Health

The word Protein is derived from the Greek word *proteios* which means 'of first importance' [1]. Whereas plant structures are primarily composed of carbohydrates, the structures of animals and humans are built on proteins [3]. Proteins function in the body in the building of new cells, the maintenance of existing cells and the replacement of old cells. In this respect proteins are the most important type of compound in the body. Proteins (as hormones) regulate metabolic processes, and (as enzymes) catalyse metabolic processes; they transport oxygen in the blood (as haemoglobin) and (as antibodies) defend the body against infection. Proteins (as nerves) transmit impulses and allow us to move by contracting our muscles. Proteins are components of skin, hair, nails and all our internal supporting tissue [1]. Another very important role of proteins is in helping to maintain the water balance in our bodies. Protein in muscles and body tissues is in a state of constant turnover, as tissue protein is degraded, nitrogen is excreted in the urine, and new protein is required daily in order to maintain the body in a stable state [3].

In addition, proteins can also be used as an emergency energy source (when there is insufficient carbohydrate). In a process called *deamination*, nitrogen is removed from the amino acids in the protein molecules, converting them to carbohydrates and rendering four calories of heat and energy per gram [1,3]. So essential is the requirement for protein that, equally in times where certain proteins may not be supplied, the body can transfer nitrogen from one amino acid to another and, if necessary, from one amino acid to a carbohydrate to manufacture a different amino acid. This process is called *transamination,* and it requires vitamin B-6 (pyridoxine) but increases the likelihood that all 20 amino acids will be used for protein synthesis [3].

Products of protein digestion are secreted into the walls of the small intestine and transported in the portal vein to the liver. The amino acids are stored in an 'amino acid pool' which is constantly changing as amino acids are added and then used by the body. The body controls and regulates the concentrations of specific amino acids and the rate at which worn and damaged muscle and organ tissue is being broken down and rebuilt from amino acids. In healthy individuals the amount of protein taken in is exactly the amount used and broken down, the excess nitrogen is excreted in faeces, urine and perspiration. This regulatory process is termed the nitrogen balance [3].

Proteins can undergo a process called denaturation, in which the unique three- dimensional structure changes. This unfolding may be slight or substantial, but the peptide bonds are not broken. When this happens, the protein ceases to function and cannot grow or change or do the work it was intended to do. In most instances, this process of denaturation cannot be reversed. Denaturation can occur to both proteins in our food and to proteins in our bodies. When this happens in the body, the results are extremely serious causing severe malfunction or sickness and could be fatal. An example of this occurs in sickle cell anaemia when the shape of the red blood cell is changed [3]. When this occurs in food products the protein "dies" in other words, it ceases to function in the way in which it was intended but can be broken down by the body to be re-used to form other proteins.

There are two considerations to maintaining the nitrogen balance; one is to do with internal conditions of health and the other with life events. Let us first deal with the internal conditions. As alluded to previously, this process of synthesising one kind of amino acid from another depends on vitamin B-6, (pyridoxine)[3]. We will come to the vitamins in the following two learning sessions, however, in the greater scheme of things without having enough vitamin B-6 (obtained from whole grain brown rice, baked potatoes, beans and bananas), our bodies have difficulty processing proteins and reconstructing worn out tissues [4]. The other thing we need is a healthy liver. The liver stores amino acids (also iron and glucose in the form of glycogen) and assists in maintaining the nitrogen balance: alcoholic liver damage results in amino acids and proteins accumulating in the liver and not being used in the body for synthesis of new proteins and tissue repair [5].

Infection, traumatic injury, pregnancy and rapid growth in infancy and early childhood increase the requirement for protein and amino acid synthesis. If this is not met, the body goes into a negative nitrogen balance, where more nitrogen is excreted than is being taken in. This, in turn, results in the body breaking down muscle tissue in order to facilitate essential repair and maintenance of the immune system in order to combat infection and prevent sepsis [3]. The problem of negative nitrogen balance and accompanying muscle wasting and lack of tissue repair and maintenance is nowhere more apparent than in those who suffer from anorexia and eating disorders [6]. Muscle mass is often equated with the circulating amino acid pool as similar quantities of muscle are destroyed and rebuilt every day. Increasing the muscle mass with resistance exercises increases the body's nitrogen turnover and its requirements, however, this also enhances the physical ability of the body to metabolise protein as well as carbohydrate [7].

Protein needs differ during different life phases. In the table of amino acids above, figures are also given for the amounts of each amino acid required for maintenance of health per kg body weight. These do not take into consideration illness or extra special requirements [3]. Although individuals will have concomitant individual requirements for proteins overall, the total protein requirement for the average adult is 0.8 grams per kg of body weight. Shortage of protein in developing countries causes kwashiorkor in infants, which is characterised by the retention of fluid in tissues alongside muscle wasting and retarded growth. A very mild form of this is evident in developed countries with the lack of quality protein in the diet where water retention in tissues, muscle weakness, and slow healing rates as well as low immune function and fatigue may be evident. The World Health Organisation (WHO) has issued a mandate that the minimum protein intake for an adult should be 23 grams [8]. As we will see in the next section, however, what you may think of as a gram of protein may, in fact, be a gram of fat or carbohydrate. We will move on now to looking at the quantity vs quality and see how we rate the quality of protein and find out how much of the protein in a given food we can use.

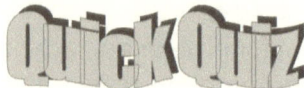

Using coloured pencils or pens place a circle around the words or labels given in the list below that you think are the ones being asked for:

1. Circle in red the functions of proteins

2. Maintaining the nitrogen balance depends on two things, circle them in blue

3. Circle in green the process by which nitrogen is removed from an amino acid

4. Circle in orange the number of calories contained in a gram of protein

5. Circle in yellow the circumstances when one needs more than the average amount of protein for one's weight

building new cells   vitamin C   pantothenic acid

digestion of food   maintaining body cells   vitamin D

repairing damaged cells   vitamin B-6   transporting oxygen

transamination   during pregnancy   catalyse

deamination   after surgery   regulating metabolic processes

twenty   twenty-three   after traumatic injury

healthy liver   four   during growth

Protein Rich Foods: Quality as Opposed to Quantity

Protein is found in most foods even if it is in only small amounts. As plants too require amino acids, there will be proteins in both plant and animal sources of foods. In general, protein makes up [9]:

> 20-36% of the weight of most pulses,
> 8-25% of nuts and seeds,
> 8-16% of whole grains.
> 10-20% of meat and fish
> 15% of eggs
> 3-4% of milk
> 1-3% of vegetables

Previously proteins were classified either as first or second class, however, today protein is classified as either of plant or of animal origin and, contrary to the older view, there is little, if any, difference between the quality of protein of animal origin from that of plant origin when the latter includes both grains and pulses. Plant protein sources provide 65% of the world food supply of edible protein of which cereals comprise 47% and pulses nuts and seeds approximately 8%. Intakes of plant protein vary little; however, intakes of animal sources of protein increases with economic prosperity [9].

Traditionally the nutritional value of proteins has been determined by their ability to provide for tissue growth [9]; protein quality has also been determined by measuring the amount of protein actually used by an organism *net protein utilisation or (NPU)*[3]. This was the simplest method of doing this whereby each food was given a particular score according to how much of the protein in it was required by the organism concerned. In more recent times, this way of determining the quality of protein has been refined as we have discovered how much of the protein in a given food is in fact digested. The WHO recognised the way of evaluating how useful a particular food is in terms of meeting our protein requirements is its 'protein digestibility corrected amino acid score (PDCAAS). Proteins that provide amino acids equal to or more than requirements receive a score of 1 (or 100%); a food with a score of 1 will meet the total protein needs of a human being during periods of growth when consumed as a sole source of protein at the minimum required rate (0.8 g/kg for adults)[3,8,10].

Some examples of the PDCAAS scores of commonly consumed foods are:

Yoghurt	1	Whole grain rye	0.68
Egg	1	Oats	0.57
Milk	1	Whole wheat	0.54
Soy	1	Lentils	0.52
Lean beef	0.92	Peanuts	0.52
Peas	0.73	Rice	0.47
Kidney beans	0.68	Corn	0.42

Protein processing and cooking methods affect the digestibility and therefore the utilisation of protein, for instance, heat treatment of milk reduces the availability of protein whilst the protein in yoghurt is pre-digested by enzymatic action resulting in the curdling of the milk, and the result is that the protein is more easily available [3]. When evaluating protein, one needs, therefore, to take the quantity of protein in a given food into consideration alongside the PDCAAS score, and the amount of processing the food has undergone. As an example:

100 g beef contains 11% protein but has a PDCAAS score of 0.92
100 g x 11% x 0.92 = 10 g of utilisable protein in 100 g of lean fillet steak

100 g soybeans contain 51% protein and have a PDCAAS score of 1
100 g x 51% x 1 = 51 g protein in 100 g dried soybeans

1 large sized 50 g egg has 15% protein and a PDCAAS score of 1
50 g x 15% x 1 = 7.5 g protein

Considering that you need 23 g protein per day which do you think is the best bet for meeting your needs?

In fact, there are other ways of meeting your needs by combining certain foods to make up the complete amino acid profile that you require. Closely related species of plants tend to make proteins of a similar amino acid profile; however very different species tend to contain a different amino acid profile. Although non-essential amino acids can be made from carbohydrate substrates, the essential amino acids are still required for this. If a food's amino acid profile does not quite match human needs, the amino acids in short supply are considered *limiting*. If a diet is based on a single plant food staple it may not foster growth due to the problem of the limiting amino acid, however, when combined with another different species of plant, the amino acid profile and protein score are considered *complementing* [3]. Cereal proteins have lower levels of the amino acids lysine and tryptophan, and pulses contain lower levels of methionine. In combination, these differences tend to cancel each other out resulting in a combination which reaches a PDCAAS score of 1[9].

Food combinations that provide all the required amino acids giving a full PDCAAS score of 1 include [3]:

Combinations	Examples
Whole grains and legumes (pulses)	Lentil biryani
	Gnushu (corn and beans)
	Bean soup and rye bread
	Bean burritos
	Dhal and rice
	Beans on whole wheat toast
	Peanut butter sandwich
Legumes (pulses) and seeds	Hummus with tahini
	Falafel
	Lentil and sesame pâté
Whole grains and dairy	Whole grain pasta and fromage frais
	Müsli and yoghurt

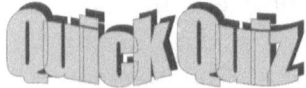

Using coloured pencils or pens place a circle around the words or labels given in the list below that you think are the ones being asked for:

1. Circle in red the good sources of proteins of vegetable origin

2. Circle in blue the good sources of proteins of animal origin

3. Circle in green the two ways of measuring the protein in food

4. Circle in orange the number of grams of protein an adult requires in a day

5. Circle in yellow food combinations that provide all the necessary amino acids

whole grain rice   NPU   thirty-seven   onion and tomato

eggs   butter beans   salmon   PDCAAS

twenty-three   pot noodles   peanut butter sandwich

tripe and onions   mushroom soup   lentil curry on rice

broccoli   yoghurt   twenty   almonds

oats   falafel in pita bread   stir fry   vegetables   ten

Combining Protein and Carbohydrate Rich Foods

Recently, and in many slimming diet books, there has been a tendency to avoid combining so-called protein foods with what is considered to be a carbohydrate or starchy foods. Diets such as the 'Beverley Hills' diet and the Fit for Life diet have maintained that certain foods are digested in different parts of the gastrointestinal system and require certain enzymes for this digestion to take place; so far so good. The fact that these enzymes are secreted in different parts of the digestive system is also correct; however, that does not necessarily mean that foods of certain origins need to be digested separately. The gastrointestinal tract is the ultimate food processor. Each day a variety of foods enters the gastrointestinal system, and with remarkable efficiency, it goes about the process of secretion of enzymes, digestion of foods and absorption of nutrients. All of this is started, regulated and stopped automatically [11].

Digestion of food is accomplished by hydrolysis under the direction of enzymes. Cofactors such as hydrochloric acid (secreted into the stomach) bile and sodium bicarbonate (secreted into the small intestine) support the digestive and absorptive processes [11]. Generally, the pH of the stomach is acid facilitating not only the digestion of proteins but also the destruction of bacteria. The pH of the small intestine is more alkaline facilitating the digestion of carbohydrate. As we have seen in this and the previous learning session, however, there are no exclusive carbohydrate or protein foods, and most foods are a combination of carbohydrates, proteins and fats as all three are essential to both animal and plant survival [3]. In essence, food is broken down and partially digested in varying degrees throughout the digestive tract [11].

The original concept of food combining began with the Hay diet based on work done by Sherman and Gettler [12] which divided foods into acid forming foods and alkali-forming foods. Potentially acid or acid ash forming foods were to be avoided in inflammatory disorders and disorders caused by or aggravated by 'over acidity'. Such foods included animal proteins, bread, baked goods, lentils and plums, prunes and cranberries. Alkali forming foods included milk and vegetables [12]. This gave rise to the old-fashioned milk and potato-based diet for gastric and duodenal ulcer patients. Science and research have now moved on, as have the techniques of correct food analysis.

Today, the combining of carbohydrate-rich and protein-rich foods has been discovered to be especially helpful in stabilising blood glucose levels and the mitigation of reactive hypoglycaemia, as well as obtaining an adequate amino acid profile and good quality protein in the diet [3]. The avoidance of acid-forming foods and a diet based on alkali-forming foods however still has some merit in dealing with inflammatory conditions such as rheumatoid arthritis and some kidney disorders. Such disorders, however, are best dealt with on an individual basis by a qualified nutritional consultant or dietician.

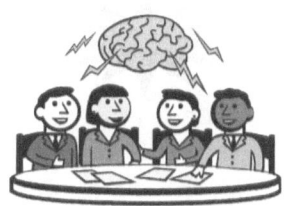

Learning Together

Learning Together

Activity 3.1: Allow yourselves 15 minutes for this activity

You will have been asked to bring a recipe with you, for between two and six people; now from your group pick one of your recipes that you would all like to work with. Between you as a group see if you can change the ingredients or the ratios of ingredients to do the following:

1. Enhance the protein in the recipe so that it gives a PDCAAS score of 1
2. Can you see a way of enhancing the micronutrient density of the recipe by changing processed ingredients for unprocessed ones or ingredients of low micronutrient nutritional density for those which are a little better?
3. Can you see a way of improving the type of fat content of this recipe?

Alternatively, for the very adventurous you might like to build a recipe from scratch!

You can add in or take away ingredients if you like and use herbs, spices and vegetable ingredients as you wish.

Write Your Notes Here

Activity 3.2: Allow yourselves 10 minutes for this activity

Now, take your own group's 'improved recipe' and swap it for another group's 'improved recipe' – look at this second recipe:

In order to improve the protein quality, quantity, or the ratio of good fats to those less beneficial, what would you:

1. Add in?
2. Take out?
3. Change?
4. Serve this dish with?

Have some fun with this, use any other ingredients such as herbs spices vegetables and fruits and see if you can make it into a 'super-improved recipe'!

Write Your Notes Here

Now you should take 5 minutes to discuss the results of your learning activities with your facilitator

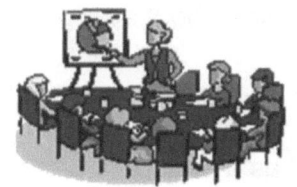

Discussion

Today's Topic for Discussion is: 'MEAT EATING VS VEGETARIANISM'

The following are two short pieces of information on some recent research. Read through these and then as a whole group we will go to the questions that follow:

Research Study 1

Three food scientists researched the nutritive value and potential health benefits of the marine crustacean krill, which has not been a traditional food in the human diet. They found that it is an abundant food source with high nutritional value and a variety of compounds relevant to human health. They thought that public acceptance of krill for human consumption would depend partly on its nutritive value. Krill is a rich source of high-quality protein, with the advantage over other animal proteins of being low in fat and a rich source of omega-3 fatty acids. Antioxidant levels in krill are higher than in fish, suggesting benefits against oxidative damage. Finally, the waste generated by the processing of krill into edible products can be developed into other value-added products [13].

Research Study 2

The effect of two diets containing different protein sources (animal vs soybean) on the low-density lipoprotein (LDL) receptor activity was tested in 12 individuals with severe type II hyperlipoproteinemia, a disorder resulting in very high cholesterol levels. The two diets, both taken for four weeks were of otherwise identical composition. During the soybean protein diet period, total cholesterol was reduced by 15.9% and LDL cholesterol by 16.4%. The diet containing animal proteins exerted no significant change in plasma lipid levels vs the baseline findings [14].

Some questions to think about as a group:

- Looking at the above, what benefits do you see as a group in using:
  - The Krill as a source of protein
  - The Soya as a source of protein
- What drawbacks do you think there might be in using:
  - The Krill as a source of protein
  - The Soya as a source of protein
- Do you think that there is any overall nutritional benefit or particular harm in being totally vegetarian?
- Do you think that there is any overall nutritional benefit or particular harm, in eating animal sources of protein daily?
- Do you think that for optimal nutrition there might be a way of compromising between animal and vegetable protein intakes?
- As a group if you think that it is possible to compromise, how would you do this?

You Might Wish to Write Some Notes Here

References

1. Sackheim GL, Lehman DD. Chemistry for the Health Sciences. 2nd ed. New York: Macmillan; 1994.
2. ACD. ACD/ChemSketch.v.10. Toronto ON: Advanced Chemistry Development Inc; 2006.
3. Ettinger S. Macronutrients: Carbohydrates, Proteins and Lipids. In: Mahan LK, Escott-Stump S (eds). Krause's Food Nutrition & Diet Therapy. 11th ed. Philadelphia: Saunders Elsevier, 2004.
4. Gallagher ML. Vitamins. In: Mahan LK, Escott-Stump S (eds). Krause's Food Nutrition & Diet Therapy. 11th ed. Philadelphia: Saunders Elsevier, 2004.
5. Baraona E, Leo MA, Borowsky SA, Lieber CS. Pathogenesis of Alcohol-Induced Accumulation of Protein in the Liver. Journal of Clinical Investigation. 1977(60):546-54.
6. Mitchell JE, Crow S. Medical complications of anorexia nervosa and bulimia nervosa. Current Opinions in Psychiatry. 2006; 19:438-43.
7. Brooks N, Layne JE, Gordon PL, Roubenoff R, Nelson ME, Castaneda-Sceppa C. Strength training improves muscle quality and insulin sensitivity in Hispanic older adults with type II diabetes. International Journal of Medical Science. 2007;4(1):19-27.
8. WHO. Energy and protein requirements report of a joint FAO/WHO/UNU expert consultation. Geneva: World Health Organisation, 1985.
9. Food, Nutrition and the Prevention of Cancer, a Global Perspective. Washington DC: World Cancer Research Fund / American Institute for Cancer Research, 1997.
10. FAO/WHO. Expert consultation on protein quality evaluation. Rome: Food and Agricultural Organisation, 1990.
11. Beyer PL. Digestion, Absorption, Transport and Excretion of Nutrients. In: Mahan LK, Escott-Stump S (eds). Krause's Food, Nutrition & Diet Therapy. 11th ed. Philadelphia: Saunders Elsevier, 2004.

12. Sherman HC, Gettler AO. The balance of acid-forming and base forming elements in food and its relation to ammonia metabolism. Journal of Biological Chemistry. 1912; 11:323.
13. Tou JC, Jaczynski J, Chen C. Krill for human consumption: nutritional value and potential health benefits. Nutrition Reviews. 2007;65(2):63-77.
14. Lovati MR, Manzoni C, Canavesi A, et al. Soy Protein Diet Increases Low-Density Lipoprotein Receptor Activity in Mononuclear Cells from Hypercholesterolemic Patients. Journal of Clinical Investigation. 1987; 80:1498-502.

LEARNING SESSION FOUR: THE FAT-SOLUBLE VITAMINS

Introduction

In this session, we will look at four of the eighteen vitamins and vitamin-like substances. The vitamins A, D, E and K are what are known as 'fat soluble', that is the intake, digestion and absorption are passive and dependent upon the dietary lipid intake. They are found in the lipid portion of the cells of the foods that contain them, such as the cell membranes or the 'germ' lipid droplets within the cell. In addition, these are the only vitamins that the body can store, again in a fatty medium. After use, they are excreted dissolved in the bile acids and passed out in the faeces. In this session, we look at these four substances, and the substances that are precursors of Vitamin A (often known as pro-vitamin A) called 'beta carotene' and cryptoxanthin, what they are, where they come from and how we can best obtain these in our diet. We discuss what they do and then move on to looking at how they work together in certain functions of our system.

We will look at our needs for these vitamins in health as well as under altered and less than ideal circumstances and the consequences of having too little and how we know when this might be the case. In addition, we look at the circumstances when we may be getting too much of one or more of these vitamins and what we need to do in these circumstances. As usual, we will have some 'quick quizzes' in between the learning sections.

After this, we go on to our two 'learning together' sessions where we will discover how much we know and can work out between ourselves. Finally, we come to our discussion and the interesting subject of taking in large doses of carotene-containing substances in the form of 'self-tanning' tablets – the pros and cons of these increasingly popular substances.

Vitamins A and E

We will deal with vitamins A and E first, especially as they tend to work together as a 'team' in some of the body's functions, predominantly those of protecting the integrity of the cell. In addition, we will discuss the two substances that are know as precursors of vitamin A or 'pro-vitamin A'. You may be able to see certain similarities in the way in which they work. We will go back in the third section to exactly how these two vitamins work together.

Vitamin A

Vitamin A is the name we use for any or all of three compounds Retinol, Retinal and Retinoic acid, also commonly referred to as 'the retinoids'. Vitamin A has a major role to play in vision, cell recognition, growth and development, the health of the immune system and the reproductive cycle. Vitamin A is an essential component of the visual pigments in the rod and cone cells that make up the retina at the back of the eye enabling light and dark adaptation and the ability for the eyes to adjust to the dark at night. Within individual cells, vitamin A affects protein synthesis within the nucleus of the cell. Although the exact mechanism is still under scientific investigation, it is known to play a role in embryonic development and in the healthy function of epithelial (skin) cells. Another important role of vitamin A is that it increases the synthesis of glycoprotein responsible for the manufacture of cell receptors that, in turn, respond to growth factors which enable cells to develop, reproduce and contributes to human growth and repair [1].

Primary deficiencies of vitamin A result from an inadequate intake [1]. Vitamin A deficiency is the most prevalent cause of blindness the world over. It is estimated that in developing countries, 250 million children are at risk [2] and between 250,000 and 500,000 cases of vitamin A deficiency-related blindness occur annually [1]. The first sign of vitamin A deficiency occurs as 'night blindness' the inability to adjust to the dark, followed by skin anomalies, such as dry bumpy skin, first noticed on the backs of the upper arms [1]. Further deficiencies result in an impaired immune function [3], breakdown of epithelial tissue in the digestive tract resulting in an inability to absorb nutrients and poor growth in the young [1,3].

Carotenoids

The Carotenoids represent the most widespread group of naturally occurring pigments in nature and are highly coloured (red and yellow) group of fat-soluble compounds. More than 600 have been discovered, but only about 30-50 are believed to have any vitamin A related activity [4]. Beta-carotene and cryptoxanthin are the two substances that are the main precursors of vitamin A, that is, that they can form vitamin A in the body [1]. Beta-carotene has been found to exhibit a higher pro-vitamin A activity [4]. Carotene supplementation seems to be a promising candidate for the alleviation of vitamin A deficiency, where gross deficiencies have caused major problems. It could be given either as a high dose capsule or through increased dietary intake. The challenge now is to improve dietary intake of vitamin A in programmes that are effective and sustainable at the community level [5].

Sources of Vitamin A and Beta Carotene

The best sources of vitamin A and Beta-carotene are contained in the red and orange pigments of food; sometimes this colouring is overlaid with chlorophyll giving the foods a dark green colour. In general, foods of animal origin contain vitamin A and those of vegetable origin Beta-carotene [1].

Food Sources of Vitamin A [1]:   Eggs

Liver

Cod liver and Halibut liver oils

Fortified milk

Food Sources of Beta-carotene [1,4]:　Pumpkin, and yellow squashes

Yellow sweet potatoes

Carrots

Peaches and apricots

Dark green leafy vegetables

Vitamin E

The fundamental role of vitamin E is to protect the body against damage from reactive forms of oxygen (*free radicals)* whether these are encountered in the environment or formed within the body because of its own metabolic processes. Substances that perform this type of action are known collectively as antioxidants. Vitamin E is, in fact, the collective name for two types of biologically active substances, the tocopherols and the tocotrienols. The tocopherols are the more active, and Dα-tocopherol is the most natural and most active form of vitamin E. Vitamin E is absorbed from foods in the upper part of the intestine, and its use depends on several factors; the dietary fat intake, the action of bile and adequate pancreatic function. Hence, the absorption of vitamin E is variable and can range from 20% to 70% of intake [1].

Vitamin E is the most important antioxidant in the human cell. It is found like vitamin A, in the lipid portion of the cell membranes and its main function is to protect the unsaturated phospholipids in the cell from damage. The process by which vitamin E does this is called *free radical scavenging*. As such, vitamin E is an important component of the cellular and thus the whole body's defence system. Vitamin E, however, does not perform this function alone and does require adequate levels of riboflavin (B2) and some of the minerals in the cell in order to function optimally [1]. Because tocopherols and tocotrienols are synthesised only by plants, plant products, especially the lipid or fatty portions of these plants, are the best sources of vitamin E. Good sources include [1]:

Almonds	Cold-pressed vegetable oils
Avocado pears	Sunflower seeds
Asparagus	Unprocessed grains
Olives	
Peanuts	

In the Western world, intakes of vitamin E is rarely low enough to cause overt deficiency diseases [6]. Because the absorption and utilisation of vitamin E depend on so many other factors, it is relatively easy to become sub-clinically deficient in vitamin E[1]. Low intakes of these antioxidant micronutrients may increase the risk of certain chronic diseases and accelerate several indicators of the ageing process. These effects may be at least partly due to inadequate protection of tissues against oxidative damage from free radicals [6]. The consequences of this manifest clinically over many years and may only be noticeable after 5 – 10 years of low grade deficiency. Changes on a cellular level are subtle and relate to damage to the system of cellular repair and renewal, signs of this are slow healing rates and faster ageing and degeneration [1].

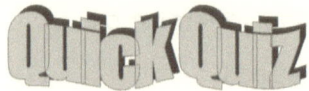

Now let's see if you can match the sources of vitamins to the given food items and combination of foods below:

Sources of vitamin A   a) _____
                                                 b) _____

Sources of Beta Carotene   a) _____
                                                 b) _____

Sources of Vitamin E   a) _____
                                                 b) _____

Sources of both vitamin A and E   a) _____
                                                 b) _____

Foods:

Liver and onions with mashed potato   Baked butternut / acorn squash

Avocado and baby spinach whole-wheat sandwich   Stuffed olives

Poached egg on whole-wheat toast   Chopped liver and Tabbouleh

Cheese and tomato omelette   Sautéed Savoy cabbage

Vitamins D and K

We will now deal with vitamins D and K which are also fat-soluble and also have one important function in common, that of building bone strength. We will take a look at how both vitamins play a role in the formation of bone tissue and the maintenance of bone health.

Vitamin D

Vitamin D is also known as 'the sunshine vitamin' as even a modest (15 minutes per day) exposure to sunlight is sufficient for the body to produce its own vitamin D from the exposure of cholesterol in the skin to ultraviolet (UV) light. This action forms the substance known as vitamin D_3 (cholecalciferol). Because D_3 can be produced in the body and acts as a 'chemical messenger' to specific target tissues it also complies with the definition of a hormone. In plants, ergosterol (a plant-based lipid) serves as a precursor to vitamin D and, when exposed to sunlight, forms Vitamin D_2. Both of these forms of Vitamin D then undergo further metabolism n the body to form *calcitriol* – the active form of vitamin D [1].

Vitamin D's most important role as calcitriol is to regulate the maintenance of the balance of calcium and phosphorous in the body, ensuring that enough calcium is carried into the bone tissue [1] (and is therefore not lining the arteries or settling into soft tissue!). In addition, Vitamin D enhances the absorption of both calcium and phosphorous from the intestines. Vitamin D, in this respect, is important in the formation of bone tissue in infants, the maintenance of bone strength and prevention of bone disorders and in the healthy formation of teeth. In times of need and when there is not enough calcium for the conduction of nerve impulses and the maintenance of blood clotting factors, Vitamin D also facilitates the recovery of calcium from the bone tissue for essential metabolic functions [1]. Scientists are still investigating other roles of Vitamin D, and it is apparent that calcitriol, the active form of this vitamin, plays a role in cell differentiation and the growth in several tissues, including skin, muscles, the pancreas, nerves, and the immune system [1,7].

Deficiency of vitamin D in early childhood results in very serious problems, the most prevalent of which is Rickets, a problem resulting in lack of mineralisation of growing bones and insufficient bone formation whilst the tendons grow normally. The bones are shortened, and the tissue is softer than it should be. Rickets results in bowed legs and ribcage 'knock knees' and the inability of bone to withstand stress and carry normal weight. Historically, Rickets has affected poor children in industrialised inner cities with malnutrition and little exposure to sunlight [1]. Today the children most at risk are dark-skinned children who are breastfed for long periods without adequate nutrition and have little exposure to sunlight [1,7]. In adults, vitamin D deficiency causes Osteomalacia which results in generalised reductions in bone density and pseudo-fractures, particularly in the spine, femur and humerus and a greater risk of fractures. Osteoporosis is a deficiency disease that results in diminished bone mass but the retention of normal bone appearance. It results from a combination of factors including deficiency of Vitamin D, impaired vitamin D metabolism due to frequent dieting, low or decreasing oestrogen levels, lack of weight-bearing exercise and ageing [1].

There are many other disorders which could result from vitamin D inadequacy and misdiagnosis of this deficiency does occur [7]. Unrecognised deficiencies of Vitamin D could reach epidemic proportions amongst some vulnerable populations [7]. In the opinion of some scientists, all persons who are dark skinned spend little time outdoors, and especially lactating mothers and their infants are at risk and could benefit from supplementation [7,8].

Vitamin D is hard to obtain in foods, and the most abundant source is controlled exposure to UV light, [1,7] however, the most prevalent sources in foods are found in [1]:

> Herring
> Salmon
> Sardines
> Chicken livers
> Shrimps
> Eggs

Vitamin K

Vitamin K is the term used collectively for three biologically active substances, phylloquinone (K_1) menaquinone (K_2) and menadione (K_3). These substances are absorbed in the intestine and, like the other fat-soluble vitamins, the process is dependent on having a minimum amount of dietary fat and on the availability of bile salts and pancreatic juices. Vitamin K has two major roles in the body one is the formation of plasma clotting carboxyglutamate (GLA) proteins which enable the clotting of blood and prevent excessive haemorrhaging from wounds. The residual compounds of the formation of GLA bind calcium, allowing it to be carried into the bone tissue [1].

Persons who do not consume enough green vegetables are at risk of vitamin K deficiency. Scientists have found that after less than two weeks of low vitamin K intake sub-clinical effects of a deficiency can be detected. Disconcertingly after dietary repletion levels of vitamin K did not return to normal several weeks later leading to the conclusion that, although a certain amount of vitamin K can be stored, this runs out fast and is hard to replace [9]. A major side effect of Vitamin K deficiency is excessive bleeding due to prolonged clotting time. Sometimes this is internal and insidious and can result in fatal anaemia [1]. New-born infants are at risk on two counts; one is the risk of haemorrhage, and prophylactic intramuscular injections of vitamin K have been found to be the most effective and safe method of preventing this problem [10]. Secondly, infants born to mothers who have been sub-clinically deficient due to low intakes of vegetables or the medicinal use of anticoagulant medication, are at risk of the bone defect chondrodysplasia punctata which results in abnormal calcification at the ends of long bones [11]. Low intakes or low absorption of vitamin K in adults is associated with increased risk of hip fractures in older adults [1].

The best food sources of vitamin K are [1]:

Spinach	Green beans
Dark leaved lettuce	Asparagus
Broccoli	Avocado pear
Dark leaved cabbage	Kale

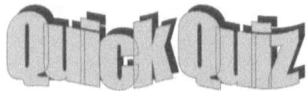

Now let's see if you can match the sources of vitamins to the given food items and combination of foods below:

Sources of vitamin D   a) _____
                                              b) _____
                                              c) _____

Sources of vitamin K   a) _____
                                              b) _____
                                            c) _____

Sources of both vitamin D and K a) _____
                                            b) _____
                                            c) _____

Foods:

Grilled Sardines with lemon and garlic   Broccoli Almandine

        Cauliflower cheese   Celery soup

Poached eggs Florentine   Salmon and cucumber sandwich

       Grilled lemon sole   Mashed carrots and swede

Mixed leaf salad   Avocado Ritz   Chicken liver pate with toast

       Fish and chips   Grilled chicken breasts

Steamed green beans with asparagus tips Hard-boiled egg salad

The Synergy Between Vitamins

Although the fat-soluble vitamins have specific functions in the body, they do not work entirely alone, and their efficacy is enhanced by a combination of factors, including having a complete profile of the support substances that are needed for the vitamins to be completely absorbed and to function optimally [1]. In this respect, vitamin A, beta-carotene and vitamin E all function as antioxidants, (along with vitamin C which we come to in the next learning session), that is, they individually protect the integrity of the cell and mitigate against damage caused by free radicals and degeneration. In this respect, they do work better together than when taken in alone.

Metabolism, like other aspects of life, involves trade-offs — oxidant by-products of normal metabolism cause extensive damage to DNA, protein, and lipid. This damage, (the same as that produced by radiation), is a major contributor to ageing and to degenerative diseases of ageing such as cancer, cardiovascular disease, immune-system decline, brain dysfunction, and cataracts. Antioxidant defences against this damage include ascorbate, (vitamin C) tocopherol (Vitamin E), and carotenoids. Dietary fruits and vegetables are the principal source of ascorbate and carotenoids and are one source of Vitamin E. Low dietary intake of fruits and vegetables doubles the risk of most types of cancer as compared to high intake and also markedly increases the risk of heart disease and cataracts [12]. Since only 9% of Americans eat the recommended five servings of fruits and vegetables per day [12] and the average British person consumes only three portions of fruit and vegetables daily with only 14% of the population consuming the recommended five portions [13], the opportunity for improving health by improving diet is great. The degenerative diseases associated with ageing include cancer, cardiovascular disease, immune-system decline, brain dysfunction, and cataracts [12].

Likewise, vitamins D and K both serve to build bones and facilitate the use of calcium. Although taking calcium supplements is justified, commonly prescribed and often recommended for older and post-menopausal women [14], the research evaluating the effect of vitamin D and calcium supplementation amongst older women in the North of England did not find much benefit to the bone density and risk of fractures [15]. This area of the country, however, is cold and gets little sunshine, older people tend not to go out too often, and the average combined fruit and vegetable consumption of this population is only 3.8 portions per day [13]. Under such circumstances, it may well be the case that inadequate amount of sunshine and not eating enough green leafy vegetables could be defeating the object!

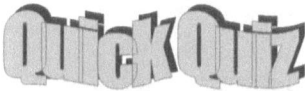

Now let's see if you can find the vitamin combinations in the foods and combination of foods below:

Foods: Vitamins:

1. Egg and avocado mixed leaf salad   _____

2. Stir fried cabbage, broccoli and almonds   _____

3. Asparagus and fresh egg mayonnaise   _____

4. Whole grain salmon salad sandwich   _____

5. Poached egg on whole grain toast   _____

6. Grilled mackerel with green beans and
    asparagus   _____

7. Roast sweet potato with wilted spinach
    and almonds   _____

8. Herring salad with fresh wild herbs, and
    olives   _____

How Much is Enough and How Much is Too Much?

Because the fat-soluble vitamins can be stored in the liver, it is possible to carry over one's day's intake into another day. In effect, this means that daily intake is not essential if one has an overall sufficiency. However, it is equally possible with high doses of these vitamins to take in too much and 'overload' the liver storage capacity which hampers the ability of the liver to perform its other functions. This does not happen when one is taking in these vitamins solely from food sources; however, it can happen when one is taking in additional supplementation with or without medical direction.

VITAMIN A AND BETA CAROTENE

Vitamin A is measured in RAE (retinol activity equivalent), 1 RAE equals the activity of 1 µg, (microgram) of retinol, which in turn is equal to 3.33 international units (IU). Beta-carotene can be converted to Vitamin A in the body, and 12 µg beta-carotene is also equivalent to 1 RAE [1]. To simplify this:

3.33 IU of vitamin A   =   1 RAE

12 µg of β-Carotene   =   1 RAE

The normal requirement:		Contained in	The upper limit:
Child	400 RAE	1 poached egg on ½ sweet potato or ½ lg cooked carrot	9000 RAE
Women	700 RAE	10 g braised lamb's liver 1 cup cooked carrots 3 fresh apricots	25,000 RAE

Men	900 RAE	15 g braised lamb's liver	28,000 RAE
		1 large baked sweet potato	
		1 cup cooked spinach + 2 eggs + ¼ cantaloupe	

Pure vitamin A can be toxic above the upper limit, which generally happens only with medication such as that given for severe acne but can also happen with overdoses of supplements of vitamin A. Toxic levels of vitamin A can cause liver dysfunction, brittle nails, hair loss, irritability and fatigue. During pregnancy overdoses of vitamin A have been known to cause birth defects [1].

VITAMIN E

Vitamin E is quantified in terms of α-tocopherol equivalents or mg α-TE. Although outdated, IU is still used on some labels for vitamin E. 1 IU = 0.67 α-TE. A daily recommended intake has been established for adults and adequate intake for infants and young children. Vitamin E is one of the least toxic of the fat-soluble vitamins, and it is virtually impossible to take in too much from food [1]. Supplements of vitamin E have been found to be safe in amounts up to 1000 α-TE (1600 IU)[6].

The normal requirement:	Contained in	The upper limit:
Child	7 mg α-TE	25 g Almonds 100 g peanuts ¼ cup raisin bran	300 mg α-TE
Adult	15 mg α-TE	1 wholegrain peanut butter sandwich +1 large avocado + 8 Asparagus spears	1000 mg α-TE

VITAMIN D

The preferred reference for vitamin D measurements is µg vitamin D_3 Still used, but in the process of being phased out are the IU equivalents, 1 µg D_3 = 40 IU. Food sources are hard to come by, and much of the intake is via conversion of sunlight on the fatty esters under the skin. High dose supplements are the most common form of toxic intake. Long-term excessive intakes leads to calcification of the soft tissues, headache, nausea, gastric upset, and in children, bone fragility and retarded growth [1].

The normal requirement:		Contained in	The upper limit:
Child	5 µg D_3	15 minutes exposure of the face, arms and hands to the sunor 50 g cooked salmon	25 µg D_3
Adult under 50	10 µg D_3	2 rollmops or 15 min sunshine or 200 g shrimp + 1 small can sardines	50 µg D_3
Adult over 50	15 µg D_3	150 g cooked salmon or 15 min sunshine + ½ can mackerel fillets or 100 g cooked halibut	50 µg D_3

VITAMIN K

There is no established dietary allowance for vitamin K, and due to the fact that it is obtained from different phylloquinones it is difficult to assess how much each would contribute to the amount of this vitamin required. The DRI (daily reference intakes) are given rather as AIs (adequate intakes) and have been estimated, as there is no means of assessing at present either how much is needed, or exactly how much food contains. There is no upper limit given at this stage. Although Vitamin K can be stored, there is no known toxicity except for accidental overdosage of injections of menaquinone. The AI can be obtained from a single portion of fruit or vegetables for a child and two portions of leafy greens for an adult, daily. If, however, digestion or absorption is compromised, a greater intake is required.

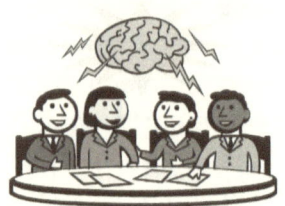

Learning Together
Learning Together

Activity 4.1: Allow yourselves 15 minutes for this activity

I think we all know the rules of this one! Find the words, forwards, backwards, diagonal and any other way you can as long as each letter is next to the previous one and the letters follow in order.

There are: 2 sources of Vitamin A and 4 sources each of Beta Carotene, vitamin D, E and K some of these foods contain more than one of these nutrients, and one food is in here twice, can you see which food this is?

WORDSEARCH

S	P	I	N	A	C	H	J	P
A	A	L	M	O	N	D	S	U
R	O	L	I	V	E	R	H	M
D	K	I	M	G	F	H	R	P
I	A	T	O	O	D	C	I	K
N	L	E	R	A	N	A	M	I
E	G	G	R	Y	E	E	P	N
S	U	G	A	R	A	P	S	A
B	R	O	C	C	O	L	I	B

Write Your Notes Here

Activity 4.2: Allow yourselves 10 minutes for this activity

4.2 a) Count up the portions of foods you ate between your group yesterday that contained the fat-soluble vitamins, or beta-carotene.

4.2 b) Take the number you arrived at and divide this by the number of people in your group to get an average for the day.

4.2 c) Taking the answer into consideration, do you think on average you received enough of these nutrients?

4.2 d) Were there any that were completely missing, or averaged at less than a full portion?

Write Your Notes Here

Now you should take 5 minutes to discuss the answers with your facilitator

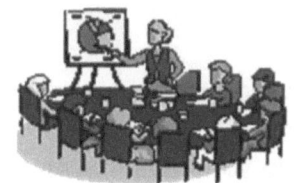

Discussion

Today's Topic for Discussion is: SELF-TANNING TABLETS, CAN THEY BE SAFE, AND DO THEY HAVE ANY BENEFITS?

Tanning tablets are generally compounds containing mainly beta-carotene 4-4-dione commonly called 'Canthaxanthin'. This substance is approved by the American Food and Drug Administration as a food colouring but is not approved for any other purpose. It is however sold as a supplement which accumulates in the skin giving it a natural looking tan [16]. Although a derivative of beta-carotene, this particular form of the substance, unlike other forms of beta-carotene, has not been found to be beneficial in the prevention of cancer [17]. In addition, researchers have found that consuming foods that are rich in carotenoids is beneficial not only in cancer prevention but in the prevention of other medical problems as well in particular heart disease, but there was no evidence that supplements proved to be better, or that the population as a whole would benefit from extra supplement intakes [18]. Canthaxanthin works by accumulating beta-carotene in the skin and other tissues as the body can only convert to vitamin A the amount of carotenoids it actually needs, any surplus is stored principally in the liver and then secondarily in the skin [19]. Although there were no reported illnesses directly resulting from the use of these tanning tablets, there is concern that there could be long-term damage from frequent use [19]. Manufacturers claim that there are benefits to taking canthaxanthin but do not cite research papers or say how they obtained this information. Tanning tablets are now no longer allowed to be sold openly in Canada as they are not considered safe; however, they are still available over the internet [16].

Some questions to think about:

- Are fair-skinned people in general overly concerned with being tanned?
- As a group do you think it is all right to take something that one feels would be of personal benefit unless and until it is proven harmful?
- Alternatively, do you think that we should err on the side of caution until we can see that such substances as tanning tablets are safe?
- Do you think that anything that colours the skin and accumulates in internal organs can really be safe in the long term?
- Although there are obvious changes, no perceived benefits but also no proven harm do you think that the use of such tablets is better than being sunburnt in the process of acquiring a tan if that is one's personal preference?

You Might Wish to Write Some Notes Here

References

1. Gallagher ML. Vitamins. In: Mahan LK, Escott-Stump S (eds). Krause's Food Nutrition & Diet Therapy. 11th ed. Philadelphia: Saunders Elsevier, 2004.
2. Wallerstein C. New sweet potato could help combat blindness in Africa. British Medical Journal. 2000; 321:786.
3. Thurnham DI. Micronutrients and immune function: some recent developments. Journal of Clinical Pathology. 1997; 50:887-91.
4. Murray MT, Pizzorno JE. Beta-carotene and Other Carotenoids. In: Pizzorno JE, Murray MT (eds). Textbook of Natural Medicine. Volume 1. St Louis: Churchill Livingstone - Elsevier, 2006.
5. Carlier C, Coste J, Etchepare M, Periquet B, Amedee-Manesme O. A randomised controlled trial to test equivalence between retinyl palmitate and beta-carotene for vitamin A deficiency. British Medical Journal. 1993;307(6912):1106-10.
6. Hathcock JN, Azzi A, Blumberg J, et al. Vitamins E and C are safe across a broad range of intakes. American Journal of Clinical Nutrition. 2005;81:736-45.
7. Holick MF. Vitamin D: importance in the prevention of cancers, type 1 diabetes, heart disease and osteoporosis. American Journal of Clinical Nutrition. 2004; 79:362-71.
8. Hollis BW, Wagner CL. Vitamin D requirements during lactation: High dose maternal supplementation as therapy to prevent hypovitaminosis D for both mother and the nursing infant. American Journal of Clinical Nutrition. 2004; 80:1752S-8S.
9. Ferland G, Sadowski JA, O'Brian ME. Dietary Induced Subclinical Vitamin K Deficiency in Normal Human Subjects. Journal of Clinical Investigation. 1993; 91:1761-8.
10. Brousson MA, Klein MC. Controversies surrounding the administration of vitamin K to newborns: a review. Canadian Medical Association Journal. 1996;154(3):307-15.

11. Vermeer C, Knapen MHK, Schurgers LJ. Vitamin K and metabolic bone disease. Journal of Clinical Pathology. 1998; 51:424-6.

12. Ames BN, Shigenaga MK, Hagan TM. Oxidants, antioxidants and the degenerative diseases of ageing. Procedures of the National Academy of Sciences. 1993; 90:7915-22.

13. The National Diet and Nutrition Survey: adults aged 19-64 years. London: Food Standards Agency, 2002.

14. Nordin BEC, Heaney RP. Calcium supplementation of the diet - justified by present evidence. British Medical Journal. 1990; 300:1056-60.

15. Porterhouse J, Cockayne S, King C, et al. Randomised controlled trial of calcium and supplementation with cholecalciferol (vitamin D_3) for prevention of fractures in primary care. British Medical Journal. 2005; 330:1003.

16. Drugs.com. Tanning Tablets Accessed 2007 10 April Drug Information Online, 2006.

17. Rosin MP. Genetic Alterations in Carcinogenesis and Chemoprevention. Environmental Health Perspectives. 1993; 101S:253-6.

18. Tribble DL, Frank E. Dietary Antioxidants, Cancer and Atherosclerotic Heart Disease. Western Journal of Medicine. 1994;161(6):605-13.

19. Sharman IM. Hypercarotenaemia. British Medical Journal. 1985; 290:95-6.

LEARNING SESSION FIVE: THE WATER-SOLUBLE VITAMINS

Introduction

The water-soluble vitamins are those of the B-complex and Vitamin C and its related substances, the bioflavonoids. These are the ones that the body cannot store, the ones that we require daily. We look at the advantages and disadvantages of this property and how to preserve the quality of foods containing the water-soluble vitamins. In addition, we look at how these substances work for us and where they are beneficial to our health. Meeting our daily needs under good conditions might not be too challenging but what about adverse conditions? We also look at when we might need more and how to meet our needs when we are not well, recovering from an illness, or surgery, or simply have ongoing altered circumstances such as pregnancy, or stressful lives and jobs. We also briefly go through the 'anti-nutrients', substances that rob us of these valuable vitamins and how they do this.

Each subsection on the B-complex vitamins and Vitamin C and bioflavonoids will also deal with the foods in which these nutrients are found and how to make the most of them. We look at what to look out for when we are shopping for them and the best way to store and cook these foods. The topic of supplements will also come up as vitamin C, in particular, has become very popular in connection with the 'common cold'.

Finally, we move on to the learning together sessions where we will engage in some fun group activities and consolidate the learning we have accomplished so far. In our general discussion for this session we will tackle the subject of 'snap; crackle and plop!' the instant packet breakfast cereals and cereal bars – are they all they're cracked up to be, or is there a let-down somewhere?

The B-Complex Vitamins

Discovered at the beginning of the 20th Century, B vitamins were originally thought to be a single substance. As nutritional science advanced, we found that they are a family of compounds all linked to various aspects of health [1]. The only thing that these vitamins have in common with vitamin C is their solubility in water and the method of absorption which is by passive diffusion across the membranes of the walls of the intestinal system. They are carried in the blood to the individual cells where they are found in the internal aqueous (watery) cellular fluid. In addition, the components of the B-complex vitamins are also different from one another, have different properties and different functions in the body. The reason they are mainly grouped together is that they are very dependent on one another as far as function is concerned. Although they have different functions within the body's cells, they are all involved as co-factors in complex metabolic functions that create energy and each individual B vitamin cannot operate properly without the other vitamins in the group also performing their individual functions [2].

As a brief reminder, these are the B-complex group of vitamins:

- B1   - Thiamine
- B2   - Riboflavin
- B3   - Niacin
- B5   - Pantothenic Acid
- B6   - Pyridoxine
- -   - Folate (Folic Acid)
- -   - Biotin
- B12   - Cobalamin

Thiamine (B1)

The basic function of thiamine is to facilitate the oxidation of glucose and function as a co-enzyme in the manufacture of Acetyl Coenzyme A (CoA) which itself is a step in the manufacture of adenosinetriphosphate (ATP) the body's energy currency. Since thiamine is essential for the oxidation of glucose, the more glucose there is in the circulation and in the cell the more thiamine one requires. Sugar and alcohol consumption tend to use up the body's thiamine resources and, in this respect, are anti-nutrients which may create a deficiency. Symptoms of mild deficiency include loss of appetite, constipation, indigestion and heaviness and weakness in the legs as well as tender calf muscles. Serious deficiency, due to dietary inadequacy and long-term and / or heavy intakes of alcohol results in the problem of beriberi, causing water retention, high blood pressure and tense calf muscles. Continuation of this problem results in *Wernicke-Korsakoff Syndrome* (Wernicke's Encephalopathy) characterised by multiple problems such as neuropathy, difficulty walking, short-term and recent memory loss, disorientation and general mental decline [2,3].

Riboflavin (B2)

Riboflavin, like thiamine, also aids in the conversion of carbohydrates as well as amino acids and lipids to energy, acting as a co-enzyme in the oxidation and reduction reactions that produce ATP within the cell. In addition to this function, riboflavin acts as an antioxidant, helping to reduce damage to the cells from free radicals and ageing [2]. Riboflavin is also required for the conversion of pyridoxine (B6) to its active form pyridoxal phosphate and a deficiency of riboflavin results in a deficiency of pyridoxine as well [2]. Deficiency of Riboflavin results in photophobia, loss of clear vision, cracked lips, greasy eruptions around the nose and a sore dark red swollen tongue as well as peripheral neuropathy [2].

Niacin (B3)

This vitamin was found in the search for the cause and cure of pellagra, a deficiency disease that devastated parts of Europe and America in the 19th and early 20th Centuries. Niacin (nicotinamide or nicotinic acid) functions as a component of the enzymes essential for all energy production in the cell, as well as being essential for cellular respiration and the synthesis of proteins and hormones within the cell. Unlike most of the B-complex vitamins, niacin is required in larger amounts of 14-18 mg per day. A deficiency of niacin results in loss of appetite, indigestion, muscular weakness and skin eruptions. Severe and long-term deficiency results in pellagra, which is characterised by dermatitis, diarrhoea, dementia, confusion, disorientation and neuropathy eventually proving fatal [2].

Pantothenic Acid (B5)

This is another vitamin that is essential in the production of CoA, the energy currency of the cell. Pantothenic acid also functions in the conversion of fatty acids to triglycerides and the synthesis of non-essential amino acids from essential ones [2]. In addition, pantothenic acid is responsible for the function of the adrenal glands and production of stress hormones [1]. Deficiencies of this substance lead to impairments in lipid synthesis, and energy production, depression, fatigue, insomnia and burning of the soles of the feet are common problems in the severely malnourished [2].

Pyridoxine (B6)

Generally, pyridoxine is the term used for several related compounds that exhibit the same functional activities, involved in the metabolism of amino acids. This substance is essential for the usage of amino acids in the formation of neurotransmitters, histamine and the precursors of haem, the protein that carries oxygen in the blood. It is also responsible for the release of glucose from stored glycogen and the biosynthesis of sphingolipids, the types of fat in the myelin sheaths that protect the nerve cells [2]. Pyridoxine is important in female hormonal balance and deficiency plays a role in PMS [1]. Deficiency symptoms of pyridoxine result in overall weakness, insomnia and peripheral neuropathy, sore tongue, mouth ulcers, and impaired immunity. Deficiencies are uncommon but often occur in conjunction with riboflavin deficiencies, and are sometimes due to medications that interfere with metabolism [2].

Folate

Folate also plays a role in the metabolism of amino acids, the conversion of essential amino acids into non-essential amino acids and in the synthesis of DNA (which plays a major role in cellular multiplication)[2]. Folate works together with vitamin B12 (Cobalamin) in the control of levels of homocysteine in the blood and consequently in reducing the risk of cardiac heart disease [4]. Folate also works with pyridoxine in the production of haem and is essential in the formation and maturation of red and white blood cells [2]. Deficiencies of folate result in impaired immunity, megaloblastic anaemia, general weakness [2], depression [5] and multiple neuropathies [2].

Biotin

Biotin is required for gluconeogenesis, the conversion of fat to glucose and subsequently energy, as well as functioning in other enzymatic and energy producing functions within the cell. The roles of biotin are linked to those of B-12, folate and pantothenic acid. Any surplus of biotin is excreted by the body within 24 hours, and this vitamin, therefore, needs to be taken in daily. It is found linked to protein-rich foods. It is required in very small amounts of approximately 30 µg per day [2].

Cobalamin (B12)

The term B12 refers to a family of Cobalamin compounds, all of which contain the mineral cobalt in the nucleus. Cobalamin plays an important role in the metabolism of amino acids and single carbon compounds and is essential for normal metabolism of all cells, in particular, those of the gastrointestinal tract, bone marrow and nervous tissue. Although only about 4 µg per day is required, a deficiency of B12 is serious, causing impaired cell division, particularly in the bone marrow and lining of the intestines. Deficiency results in both megaloblastic anaemia, and pernicious anaemia resulting in neurological abnormalities with nerve demyelination. Symptoms include numbness and burning of the feet, stiffness and general weakness of the legs. A common cause of deficiency is lack of the Intrinsic Factor (IF) in the stomach that is necessary for the absorption of B12 [2]. In addition, B12 is the only B vitamin that can be stored for a period of time; however, it is only available from animal products, and persons who are consuming a diet based solely on foods of vegetable origin will become deficient over a period of 5-6 years [2]. It has been a common belief over the years that fermented foods contain B12; however, this has now been refuted by scientific investigation [2].

Meeting One's Needs for the B-Complex Vitamins

The adult requirement of most of the B-complex vitamins is between 1 and 2 mg per day, although somewhat larger amounts of niacin (14-18 mg) and pantothenic acid (4-5 mg) are required. A summary of which foods contain the best sources of the B-complex vitamins is given here:

Food	Vitamins
Unprocessed cereals,	Thiamine, Riboflavin, Niacin, Pantothenic acid
Pork – lean trimmed	Thiamine, Biotin, B12
Beef – liver	Riboflavin, Biotin, B12
Tuna fish	Niacin, Biotin, B12
Mushrooms	Niacin, Pantothenic acid
Sweet potatoes	Pantothenic acid
Nuts, sunflower seeds	Niacin
Pulses, broccoli and leafy green vegetables	Pantothenic acid, Folate

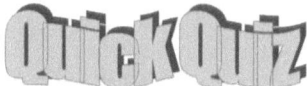

Can you tell the myths and 'old wives tales' about vitamin B-complex from the scientific facts?

<u>Myth or Fact?</u>

1. You can get vitamin B12 from potato skins   _____

2. Yeast extract is a good source of vitamin B-complex   _____

3. The B-complex vitamins are interdependent and work together   _____

4. The main function of many of the B vitamins is to produce energy within the body's cells   _____

5. You can go for months without consuming B vitamins as they can be stored   _____

6. A high consumption of sugar enhances the body's utilisation of thiamine, thereby giving you more energy   _____

7. Niacin was discovered in the search for the cause and cure for pellagra, which can be fatal   _____

8. Wernicke Korsakoff Syndrome is due to a deficiency of thiamine, excessive alcohol intake increases the risk   _____

9. The requirement for B-complex vitamins is small and deficiencies are unlikely, regardless of health and age   _____

10. Cobalamin and Pyridoxine both play a vital role in the metabolism of amino acids   _____

Vitamin C and the Bioflavonoids

Vitamin C (the chemical name is Ascorbic Acid) can be synthesised by plants from glucose and many carnivorous animals from glucose and galactose, however, human beings are among the exceptions. For us, therefore, this vitamin is not only a necessity, but it is also essential in that it must be consumed in food form daily. Vitamin C has so many functions it is difficult to know how the body could possibly manage without it and research into its uses in the body is still very much ongoing [2]. One of the primary functions of Vitamin C is its involvement in the formation of collagen, a protein which is the substance that holds cells of the skin, cartilage, tendons, bone matrix and tooth dentin together [6]; as well as carnitine, which is essential for the oxidation of fatty acids [2]. In addition, it is responsible for the utilisation of steroid hormones produced by the adrenal glands and works in conjunction with vitamin A, beta-carotene and vitamin E as an antioxidant [2]. In this latter respect, it has an important function in protecting the body against damage from free-radicals [6]. Dietary vitamin C is an indispensable component of the antioxidant matrix, like vitamins A, E and beta-carotene function to quench free radicals in the fatty components of the cell, vitamin C functions in the watery aqueous medium acting as a potent free radical scavenger inside the cell itself [7].

Another major function of vitamin C is the production of interferon which is the body's own destroyer of rogue cells and its involvement with the leucocytes, white blood cells that destroy bacteria and viruses. In these respects, it promotes resistance to infection. In addition, vitamin C also helps to maintain good lung function and prevent respiratory diseases [2]. Vitamin C also aids in the absorption of non-haem iron (iron from vegetable sources), and in this respect prevents iron-deficiency anaemia in vegetarians [6].

Acute deficiency of vitamin C is scurvy and signs of this can be seen after 45-60 days of vitamin C deprivation. In children, the syndrome is called Moeller-Barlow disease, and it occurs in infants fed on a formula which is not enriched with vitamin C. Signs of deficiency in both children and adults include impaired wound healing, oedema, haemorrhages due to capillary breakdown, and weaknesses in bone, cartilage, teeth and connective tissue. Adults may have swollen bleeding ulcerated gums and tooth loss, in addition to lethargy, fatigue and changes in psychological function including hysteria, hypochondria and depression [2].

The bioflavonoids have no known individual metabolic function; however, when taken with vitamin C they enhance its function, reducing capillary fragility and potentiating the antiscorbutic activity of vitamin C. Studies have shown a relationship between diets high in the bioflavonoids and reduced risks for cardiovascular disease and certain cancers. The main bioflavonoids that are known to be active are rutin, hesperidin and quercetin, which are the major sources of non-carotenoid red, blue and yellow pigments in plant foods [2].

Infants and children require 30 mg vitamin C daily, and adults require, between 75 and 120 mg. The average orange contains 60 mg, and the average cigarette uses up 25 mg! Dietary fruits and vegetables are the principal sources of vitamin C [8]. The following is a list of foods which contain both vitamin C and bioflavonoids [2]:

Oranges	Tomatoes
Blackberries	Sweet red and yellow peppers
Strawberries	Broccoli (particularly purple headed)
Cantaloupe	Brussels sprouts
Mango	Kale

Normal Requirements and Extra Requirements

Although the B-complex vitamins are required in relatively small amounts, many people have minor sub-clinical deficiencies, sometimes from an inadequate food intake but often from an enhanced requirement [4]. Life does not always run smoothly, and neither does our requirement for nutrients, particularly the water-soluble vitamins. We may require more than the normal intake in times of growth, such as pregnancy and, in times of recovery from certain illnesses, or the need for preventing illnesses [1,2]. During pregnancy, an increased intake of folate has been linked with a decrease in neural tube defects in newborns [2] and in the alleviation of post-partum depression [1]. Sub-optimal intakes that do not cause outright disease but increase the risk of disease may be more common than we think, the elderly being especially prone [4]. Increases in folate have also been linked with decreases in colon cancer, and cervical dysplasia [1] and persons with low thyroid function may have an increased need for riboflavin [1]. Niacin has been found to be beneficial in Reynaud's disease and in the maintenance of glucose levels in type 2 diabetes [1].

Vitamin C is the most common supplement taken in the US [9] and possibly other Westernised countries as well. There has been controversy surrounding vitamin C and the common cold, however, a review of research trials revealed that there was no difference in the number of colds when taking high doses of vitamin C. Findings did reveal that 250 mg per day of vitamin C shortened the duration of colds and reduced the severity of symptoms in those who were extremely active outdoors and more vulnerable to respiratory diseases [10]. Dietary fruits and vegetables are the principal sources of vitamin C and evidence suggest that diets high in vitamin C have a cancer-protective effect [9]. Although evidence for supplementation of vitamin C is not conclusive, supplementing is not at all unsafe and intakes of up to 2 000 mg are generally well tolerated, the only side effect of extremely high doses being diarrhoea which ceases as soon as the supplementation is halted [11]. Supplementation may be beneficial for vulnerable groups of people and especially for those who smoke. The WHO have promoted national nutritional policies for chronic disease prevention [12] and food fortification with vitamins and risk group supplementation may be vital in the prevention of long-term chronic disease [13].

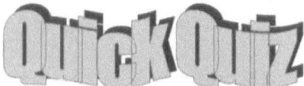

Can you tell the myths and 'old wives tales' about vitamin C and bioflavonoids and meeting our needs from the scientific facts?

<u>Myth or Fact?</u>

1. Some animals have the ability to synthesise vitamin C from glucose and galactose

    _____

2. Vitamin C is not essential for humans, but it helps to prevent disease if we have a reasonable amount

    _____

3. No matter how much vitamin C you take in it makes no difference to the health of bones, and teeth

    _____

4. Vitamin C promotes resistance to infection

    _____

5. Bioflavonoids can replace vitamin C in the diet

    _____

6. Strawberries don't have many nutrients, it's the cream that counts for something!

    _____

7. After less than two months without vitamin C the signs of scurvy are likely to be visible

    _____

8. Moeller-Barlow disease occurs in infants fed on formula that lacks vitamin C

    _____

9. Bioflavonoids can enhance the function of vitamin C

    _____

10. A single orange contains enough vitamin C for an adult even if they smoke

    _____

Preserving 'Vulnerable' Vitamins in Food

The processing of food and drinks including preservation and preparation is a defining characteristic of civilisation. Preservation and cooking of food are tasks and pleasures as well as an intrinsic and defining part of the worlds varied cultures [6]. The processing of foods by any means alters their structure and the content and availability of nutrients. To a large extent the fat-soluble vitamins, are less easily destructible as they are preserved in the cell walls of the fatty parts of the molecules in the foods in which they are found. That is not to say they are indestructible, but that they are less vulnerable to destruction by light, heat and storage. The water-soluble nutrients, however, are highly vulnerable to heat, light and cooking methods.

Grains are usually milled, and for the main part, all or some of the outer bran layer is removed, except for rice which is usually refined (de-husked, and polished to remove the outer layer). In general, most starches are cooked before they are eaten [6]. Wheat is mainly de-husked, the germ containing the vitamin E is often removed along with the bran, and the wheat is milled and cooked and consumed in the form of bread, pasta and other white flour products. Corn is also de-pitted, removing the germ containing the vitamin E. Although the consumption of starches in Westernised countries has decreased from an original 70% of the diet down to between 22 and 40%, what is still consumed is mainly refined [6]. The result is that Vitamin E and non-starch polysaccharide (fibre) intake from these sources may be insufficient and B-complex intake marginal. Refrigeration preserves the value of foods without the need for salting, curing or smoking, all of which are less beneficial to one's health. Refrigeration delays spoiling and microbial contamination and, in particular, prevents fats from becoming rancid, thus preserving fat soluble nutrients [6].

Cooking of food is probably the most common way of both preserving and consuming foods in general. Some cooking methods are, however, better than others. The water-soluble vitamins are greatly reduced when using water and heat. Vitamin

C is also destroyed by light and any form of UV radiation. As far as temperature is concerned [6]:

Steaming, boiling and stewing	heat does not exceed 100 °C
Microwaving (short time period)	heat may go up to 200 °C
Baking and roasting (longer time)	heat may go up to 220 °C
Grilling broiling and barbecue	heat may go up to 400 °C
Frying	heat may go up to 450 °C

In general, the less heat and water used the better the vitamin preservation. Steaming, stewing and quick bursts of microwaving (without water) preserve more nutrients than other forms of cooking. However, the author acknowledges the fact that the use of microwaves in food preparation over the longer term is controversial and may be under-researched. If food is boiled, one should avoid discarding the water and rather use it for sauce or soup as many nutrients will have leached into the water that could be consumed. Light, as well as heat, diminishes the vitamin C content of foods considerably, so it is better if foods rich in vitamin C are stored in dark containers, kept in brown paper bags, or refrigerated. When shopping for food, it is best to:

- Buy grains as unprocessed as possible
- Purchase fruits and vegetables as fresh as possible and store away from heat and light
- Do not peel fruit and vegetables before use
- Do not cut up fruit, or juice it, and leave it in a clear container
- Buy fruit juice in dark bottles, or cartons, and refrigerate
- Cook vegetables quickly in a minimum of water, do not use soda to preserve colour as this destroys the vitamins
- When cooking grains:
  - Wash well
  - Use one-part grain to two parts cold filtered water
  - Bring just to the boil, turn down heat to a minimum, cover and cook until all water is absorbed and do not rinse

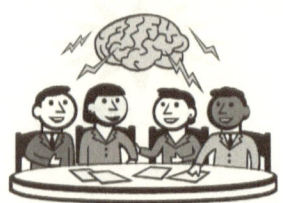

Learning Together
Learning Together

Activity 1: Allow yourselves 10 minutes for this activity

In your groups match the foods to the nutrients or groups of nutrients given below to ensure that all the vitamins you need in any given day are included:

Food   Vitamins

Oranges   _____

Whole-grain Bread   _____

Lean Roast Ham   _____

Bowl of Leafy Salad   _____

Green Beans   _____

Eggs   _____

Carrots _____

Avocado _____

Salmon _____

Beta Carotene & K   D & E   Biotin and B12   E & A

K   C & Bioflavonoids   Thiamine & Riboflavin Folate

C & E   A   B12 & Folate   E   Riboflavin

Thiamine, Niacin, Riboflavin & Pantothenic Acid   Folate and A

Beta Carotene   K & E   D & Omega 3   C & Omega 6   Riboflavin

<u>Write Your Notes Here</u>

Activity 2: Allow yourselves 15 minutes for this activity

Please try to fill the grid with foods in such a manner that every row, every column and every 3 x 3 box accommodates all the foods one needs in a given day to provide all the vitamins one requires without repeating any.

Vitamin Sudoku

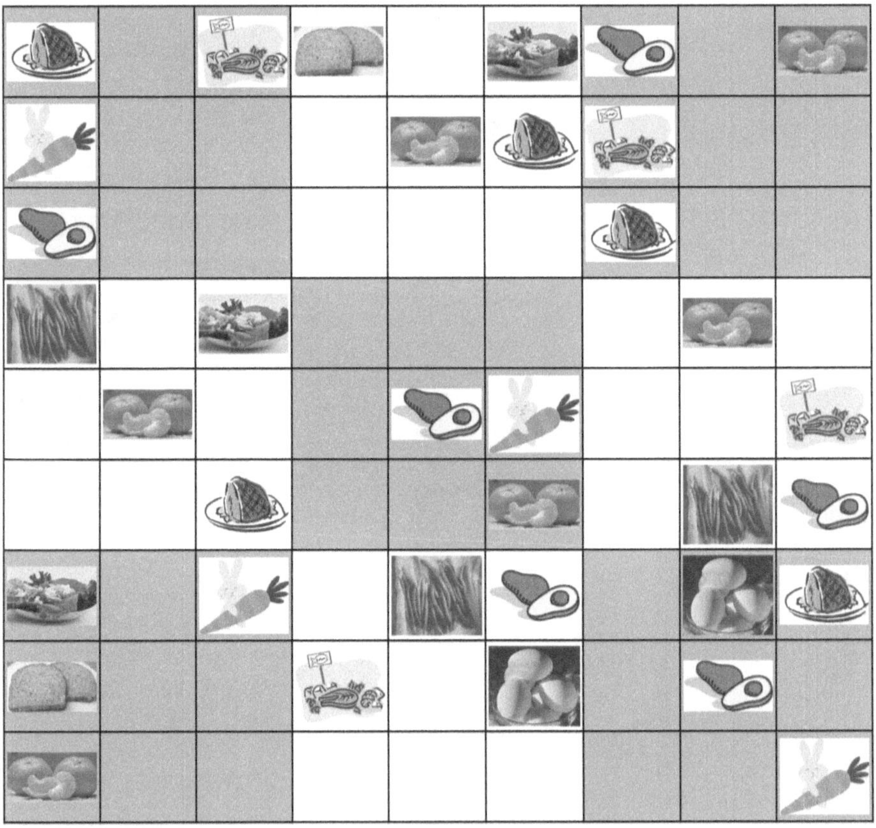

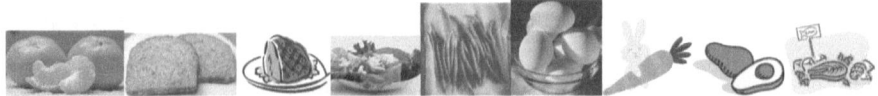

© A. A. Morris-Paxton 2019

<u>Write Your Notes Here</u>

Now you should take 5 minutes to discuss the answers with your facilitator

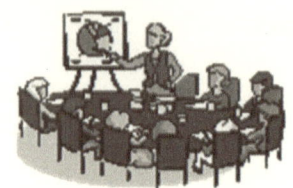

Discussion

Today's Topic for Discussion is: INSTANT BREAKFAST – SNAP CRACKLE AND PLOP?

In research to assess the sales of various segments of the ready to eat breakfast cereal market after an advertising campaign, researchers found that after a big advertising campaign, endorsed by the national cancer institute (NCI) (USA) that promoted high fibre cereals, growth was achieved at the expense of cereals that were not promoted as high fibre but were nonetheless whole-food[14]. The same company also promoted a cereal bar version of the product. In addition, cereal bars in themselves have become a popular alternative to breakfast. The Author looked at the contents of one highly promoted cereal, one non-promoted cereal and a popular low fat, low-calorie breakfast bar:

<u>Contents of Promoted High Fibre Cereal:</u>

Wheat Bran	85%
Sugar	15% All other ingredients together

Barley Malt (a form of sugar)
Flavouring
Glucose-Fructose Syrup (a form of sugar)
Salt and added vitamins: Thiamine, Folate, Vitamin D, B12

<u>Contents of Non-Promoted Cereal:</u>

Wholegrain Oats	88%
Sugar	6.8%
Pre-biotic Oligosaccharides	5.2%

Salt and added vitamins: Thiamine, Riboflavin, Niacin, Folate, Iron

Contents of Breakfast Bar

Cereals (Wheat Oats and Rice)	52%
Pre-biotic Oligosaccharides	29%
Fruit Juice Concentrate	9%
Dried Apple Pieces	4%
Sweetened cranberries	1.7%
Freeze Dried Raspberry	1%
Sugar, Salt Flavourings, Preservatives and Milk Solids make up other	3.3%
Total calories	70

Some questions to think about and discuss with the whole group:

- Do you think that even approved advertising campaigns that are perceived to be promoting healthy foods are all together truthful?
- Do you think that you can always trust 'approval badges' on the packaging such as 'Heart Foundation' or 'NCI Approved'?
- Do you think that you can afford not to read the labels?
- How does the group think that one might overcome the problem of labels being difficult to read, too small print or using scientific terms and names of ingredients that the ordinary person might not understand?
- What effects do you think that shopping in a hurry or while harassed with small children have on what you buy?
- As a group, how do you think that you can counter the effects of advertising that is not always to your advantage?

<u>You Might Like to Make Some Notes Here</u>

References

1. Kreloff J. B-Complex Vitamins - Powerful Healing Nutrients. Boulder: Design for Health Institute, 2001.
2. Gallagher ML. Vitamins. In: Mahan LK, Escott-Stump S (eds). Krause's Food Nutrition & Diet Therapy. 11th ed. Philadelphia: Saunders Elsevier, 2004.
3. Becker CE. Alcohol and Drug Use - Is There a Safe Amount? Western Journal of Medicine. 1984; 141:884-90.
4. Fletcher RH, Fairfield KM. Vitamins for Chronic Disease Prevention in Adults. Journal of the American Medical Association. 2002;287(23):3127-9.
5. Abou-Saleh MT, Coppen A. Folic acid and the treatment of depression. Journal of Psychosomatic Research. 2006(61):285-7.
6. Food, Nutrition and the Prevention of Cancer, a Global Perspective. Washington DC: World Cancer Research Fund / American Institute for Cancer Research, 1997.
7. Tribble DL, Frank E. Dietary Antioxidants, Cancer and Atherosclerotic Heart Disease. Western Journal of Medicine. 1994;161(6):605-13.
8. Ames BN, Shigenaga MK, Hagan TM. Oxidants, antioxidants and the degenerative diseases of ageing. Procedures of the National Academy of Sciences. 1993; 90:7915-22.
9. Donaldson MS. Nutrition and Cancer: A Review of the Evidence for an Anticancer Diet. Nutrition Journal. Volume 3, 2004.
10. Hemila H, Chalker E, D'Souza R, Douglas R, Treacy B. Vitamin C for preventing and treating the common cold. The Cochrane Database of Systematic Reviews. Volume 4, 2004.
11. Hathcock JN, Azzi A, Blumberg J, et al. Vitamins E and C are safe across a broad range of intakes. American Journal of Clinical Nutrition. 2005; 81:736-45.
12. WHO. Diet, Nutrition and the Prevention of Chronic Diseases: Report of a Joint WHO/FAO Expert Consultation. Geneva: World Health Organisation, 2003.

13. Tulchinsky TH, Kaluski DN, Berry EM. Food fortification and risk group supplementation are vital parts of a comprehensive nutrition policy for prevention of chronic diseases. European Journal of Public Health. 2004;14(3):226-7.
14. Levy AS, Stokes RC. Effects of a Health Promotion Advertising Campaign on Sales of Ready-To-Eat Cereals. Public Health Reports. 1987;102(4):396-403.

LEARNING SESSION SIX: THE MINERALS

Introduction

In this session, we look at the 'Cinderella' of nutrition – the minerals. These are the small, non-organic, often forgotten and incredibly hard-working components of our nutritional profile that seem to get ignored, yet without which we would not exist! There are a total of 18 essential minerals which are inorganic elements as opposed to organic molecules, often present in ionic form in our bodies. There are two groups of minerals; those we need more of (the macrominerals, also known as the electrolytes), which keep the fluid balance and neuromuscular function stable and those we need in very tiny amounts, the microminerals or trace elements, which do a host of other small, but vital, jobs in our body.

We will begin with the macrominerals and their functions. Deficiencies of macrominerals are rare, but imbalances can lead to serious problems which we will highlight. We then go on to the microminerals and their functions, before looking at ways in which we can obtain all the elements that we need in the correct amounts from our foods. We discuss which foods contain the best sources of these nutrients, how to conserve them in cooking and what to look out for in order not to create a mineral imbalance.

We then come to our learning together sessions where we have some fun with our newly acquired knowledge, and finally we end with our discussion topic for the session. There appears to be a strong link between salt intake and hypertension (high blood pressure); however some scientists feel that this link is not enough to warrant an overall restriction of salt for the public. However, the cost of hypertension is rising, and some nutritionists feel we are doing too little too late when it comes to dealing with this major problem. We look at this issue in today's discussion and ask a few thought-provoking questions.

The Macrominerals and Electrolytes

Minerals represent between 4% and 5% of total body weight. Approximately 50% of the mineral content of the body is calcium and, 25% is phosphorous which exists in the form of phosphates. Most of these two elements are found in bones and teeth. The five other essential macrominerals, magnesium, sodium, potassium, chloride and sulphur and the eleven established microminerals make up the other 25% of the body's mineral content. The macrominerals are those we need in larger amounts of 100 mg per day or more. These exist in the body and in food mainly in the ionic state, (except for sulphur) and form positive ions (cations); however, they also exist as compound salts such as sodium chloride and calcium phosphate, or as components of organic compounds. Bioavailability has become a useful term to describe the state of minerals within the lumen of the small intestine. With the exception of haem iron (iron which is obtained from meat) the minerals are found and absorbed in the ionic state, that is those which are still bound in a compound form to some other organic or inorganic substance, after the process of digestion, are not absorbed, i.e. they are not bioavailable and are eliminated through the bowels [1].

Once minerals have passed through the intestinal lumen, they must still be transported around the body which requires an active transport mechanism, especially for the cations. Thus the bioavailability of some minerals is quite low, and this may have been originally an evolutionary mechanism to reduce the possibility of toxicity from an overabundant intake of some minerals [1].

Calcium

Calcium is the most abundant mineral in the human body and, by itself, makes up between 1.5% and 2% of the total body weight, 99% of which is contained in the bones and teeth. The minerals in the teeth are fixed by the time they erupt and are 'non-returnable'. The calcium and other minerals in the skeleton, however, can be mobilised back into the bloodstream for delivery to the tissues, if necessary, in times of shortage or extra need [1]. Later in life, the absorption of calcium from the blood into the bones is limited unless it is accompanied by adequate vitamin D; however, the bone continues to give up calcium when required, and calcium continues to be lost via the faeces and urine. Urinary calcium losses rise with menopause. Hence the bones are at risk for thinning and the development of osteoporosis in later years [2]. The remaining 1% of calcium is in the blood, extracellular fluids and within the cells of all tissues, where it has some important functions. The transport functions of cell membranes are influenced by calcium as is the transmission of ions across the cell membranes [1]. Calcium is also needed for the neurotransmitters which send messages along the nerve pathways and the contraction and relaxation of muscles. It is one of four minerals (the others being sodium, potassium and magnesium) especially important in the regulation of heart muscle function. A significant increase in the blood calcium level can cause respiratory failure, and a significant decrease can lead to tetany of the skeletal muscles. Calcium is also important for the clotting of blood [1].

Phosphorous

Phosphorous, after calcium, is the next most abundant mineral in the human body with on average 700 g being contained in the body, 85% of which is found in the bones and teeth, the remaining 15% being present in the cells of all the remaining tissues, including the extracellular fluid. Generally, the efficiency of phosphate absorption is 60-70% in a healthy adult, the remainder being excreted in the urine. Chronic undernutrition, increases in plasma insulin and other metabolic disturbances all result in low phosphate levels as well as increased losses of phosphorus in the urine. Phosphorous contributes to numerous cellular functions, including the generation of energy within the cell, healthy cell division and formation of the nucleus of new cells and the prevention of acidosis and, most importantly, the formation of teeth and bones. Phosphate deficiency is rare but occurs in persons taking phosphate binding medications over a long period of time. Intakes are lower in strict vegetarians, and retention is lower in the elderly. Severe deficiency results in extreme fatigue and neural, skeletal, renal and muscular dysfunction. In extreme cases, this can be fatal [1].

Magnesium

After potassium, magnesium is the second most abundant cation within the cells of the body. The adult body contains between 20 g and 28 g of magnesium, 60% of which is found in the bones, 26% in muscle tissue and the rest in the other body organs and body fluids. About 35% - 45% of the magnesium taken in is absorbed, and excess is excreted in the urine. Magnesium is required for over 300 enzymatic reactions in the body necessary for the metabolism of food components. In addition, magnesium works together with calcium in muscle contraction and relaxation and acts as a physiological calcium channel blocker in cardiac function. High magnesium intakes are associated with greater bone density; however, many people in Westernised countries are slightly deficient in magnesium, resulting in muscular spasms, and a tendency towards blood clotting [1]. Magnesium intake has been found to be related to the control of blood lipid levels and the genesis of atherosclerosis (hardening of the arteries), with low intakes of magnesium increase the risk of arterial damage [3]. Severe deficiency results in tremors, muscle spasms, personality changes, anorexia, nausea and vomiting and leads eventually to tetany and convulsions if left unchecked [1].

Sulphur

Although technically a mineral, sulphur is a component of organic molecules and exists in the body as a constituent of three amino acids, cystine; cysteine, and methionine [1]. It functions entirely as an organic molecule and is taken in the diet only as a part of the essential amino acids cysteine and methionine [4]. Groups of sulphur containing proteins function as part of various cellular reactions and are a component of heparin, a protein which prevents inappropriate clotting of blood, and chondroitin sulphate, itself a component of cartilage and bone. Both excesses and deficiencies are unlikely [1]. Requirements for macrominerals:

Mineral	Minimum Daily Requirements	Maximum Daily Recommended	Obtained From:
Calcium	1,200 mg	2,500 mg	Dark green leafy vegetables; broccoli; sardines; canned salmon; soybeans, yoghurt
Phosphorous	700 mg	4,000 mg	Fish; eggs; yoghurt; nuts; seeds, legumes
Magnesium	320 mg	350 mg	Seeds; nuts; legumes; whole grains; green vegetables
Sulphur	–	–	Protein-rich foods (especially eggs); garlic

The Electrolytes

Simply explained, the electrolytes are substances that, when dissolved in water, dissociate into positive (cations) and negatively (anions) charged ions. They exist as either simple inorganic salts of sodium, potassium or magnesium, or as complex organic molecules. Three indispensable dietary constituents, sodium, potassium and chloride, commonly known as *the electrolytes,* are related and their functions are inseparable. Potassium constitutes 5%, chloride 3% and sodium 2% of the total mineral content of the body. These elements together are distributed throughout the body's fluids and are involved in maintaining four very important functions [1]:

- Water balance and distribution
- Osmotic equilibrium in the cell
- Acid-base (alkali) balance within the body
- The correct concentration of intracellular and extracellular fluids and minerals

Sodium

Sodium is the major cation (Na^+) in the extracellular fluid (the water and dissolved substances in the spaces outside the cell). 30-40% of the body's sodium is bound in the bones and is not exchangeable. Contrary to popular belief, there is very little sodium lost in perspiration. The normal serum sodium concentration is expressed in mEq/L and is 136-145 mEq/L. The main function of sodium is the regulation of the volume of extracellular fluid; it also aids in the conduction of nerve impulses and the control of muscular contraction. Most of the sodium losses are through urine with minimum amounts lost through the bowels and perspiration. The kidneys filter sodium from the blood and retain and pump back into the system the amount required for function, in this way preserving sodium and preventing a net loss [1].

Chloride

Chloride (Cl^-) is the principal anion of extracellular fluids, the highest concentration being found in the cerebrospinal fluid, bile and gastric and pancreatic juices. In the stomach, chloride is secreted by the gastric lining as hydrochloric acid, which provides an acid medium for digestion (particularly the digestion of proteins) and the activation of digestive enzymes. Chloride, in addition to sodium, also helps to maintain water balance and osmotic pressure and is crucial to maintaining the balance between acid and alkali in the body. Chloride is absorbed in the small intestine and excreted in the urine and in perspiration. Chloride losses parallel sodium losses but are greater with the use of diuretics, or vomiting [1]. Our major source of chloride comes like sodium from table salt (sodium chloride), however, as all green plants contain chloride (this is what gives them their green colour), it is also possible to acquire this mineral from vegetable matter without the intake of table salt [1].

Potassium

Potassium is the major cation (K^+) of intracellular fluid and is present in extracellular fluid only in small amounts. The major function of potassium is to maintain normal water balance, osmotic equilibrium and the acid-alkali balance of the body. In addition to calcium, it is important in the regulation of neuromuscular function and promotes cellular growth. As the potassium content of muscle tissue is related to muscle mass, extra potassium is required during periods of muscle growth. Potassium is absorbed from the small intestine and excreted via the urine, a process controlled by the kidneys.

Requirements for electrolyte minerals:

Mineral	Minimum Daily Requirements	Maximum Daily Recommended	Obtained From:
Sodium	200 mg	2,400 mg	Meat; chicken; fish; eggs; dairy produce; sodium chloride as table salt
Chloride	750 mg	Not known	Green vegetables; table salt
Potassium	2,000 mg	3,500 mg	Fruits; vegetables; nuts; dairy produce

Avoiding Problems of Electrolyte Imbalance

Although deficiencies of the electrolyte minerals are rare, imbalances are common and can cause problems with fluid balance and acid/base balance provoking further medical complications [1]. Sodium deficiency generally occurs only in conjunction with the loss of other minerals due to excessive vomiting and / or severe diarrhoea [5]. This is in part due to the imbalanced intake of minerals which is contrary to what the human physiology was originally designed to deal with. Physically the body is very capable of conserving sodium, but not potassium, as sodium until recently was hard to come by! The bulk of the original diet was rich in potassium and poor in sodium as it consisted mainly of wild herbs, roots, shoots, berries, fruits and wild grains with occasional fresh meat and fish as and when available [6].

The mean daily dietary salt intake in Western societies is 10-12 g (4 -5 g sodium) which is far and above the minimum requirement and twice the maximum recommended daily intake [1]. The most common source of sodium is table salt, not only that which is added at the table but also in cooking, prepared foods, takeaway foods and restaurant meals, as well as both sweet and savoury snacks, baked goods and breakfast cereals. Protein-rich foods such as meat, eggs and dairy products contain more naturally existing sodium, whereas vegetables contain very little and fruit little or none [1].

Whereas even an isolated excessive intake leads to oedema and hypertension, the kidneys can deal with this by excreting more sodium over a period of time, thus correcting a temporary imbalance and reversing the symptoms. Consistent excessive sodium intake is, however, of primary concern [1]. This is exacerbated by the concomitant low intake of potassium, thus creating an imbalance of the ratios of sodium to potassium that is contrary to what the human physiology was designed to deal with. The resulting problems include:

- Hypertension, leading to cardiovascular disease and stroke [7-10]
- Decreased bone mass, leading to osteoporosis [6,9]
- Formation of kidney stones [9,11]
- Oedema (water retention) [1,8]

Avoidance of these problems will require a change back to taking in more potassium than sodium. Measures to facilitate this include:

- Increasing the intake of fresh fruits and vegetables to a minimum of five portions but a recommended intake of 5-9 portions per day [6,8,12,13]
- Increasing the intake of whole grains and pulses [6,8]

- Eliminating additional table salt and decreasing the intake of pre-prepared meals containing salt [6,8]
- Decreasing the intake of meats and dairy products (especially full fat and processed dairy foods) [6,8]

The benefits of restructuring the diet not only mitigate the problems of excessive sodium intake but, by increasing the dietary potassium concomitantly, facilitate better use of other minerals and increase the amount of dietary antioxidants and vitamins. This has other benefits and, not only protects against hypertension, stroke and osteoporosis but also many forms of cancer [14]. The increased intake of potassium facilitates better neuromuscular function and the generation of lean muscle tissue [1].

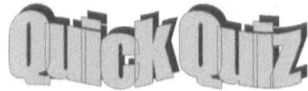

1. The minerals that play the biggest role In water balance are:

   Answer: _____

   A. Potassium, Magnesium and Sodium

   B. Potassium, Calcium and Sulphur

   C. Sodium, Chloride and Potassium

   D. Phosphorous, Sodium and Potassium

2. The macrominerals that contribute the most to bone development are:

   Answer: _____

   A. Potassium, Calcium and Phosphorous

   B. Calcium, Phosphorous and Magnesium

   C. Calcium Magnesium and Sulphur

   D. Potassium, Calcium and Magnesium

3. The most abundant mineral in the human body is

   Answer: _____

   A. Sodium

   B. Phosphorous

   C. Calcium

   D. Magnesium

4. Most of the body's mineral content is found in

   Answer: _____

   A. The bones

   B. The blood

   C. The muscles

   D. The kidneys

5. The best source of chloride is found in

   Answer: _____

   A. Recycled tap water

   B. Bottled mineral water

   C. Table salt

   D. Green vegetables

The Microminerals

There are numerous elements present in body tissues in minute amounts that have been found to be essential for optimal health, growth and development. These are known as the *microminerals*, often termed *trace elements*. As with the macrominerals, each one has its own niche in the optimum function of the human being and a range of functions that depend much upon the dosage taken in and the overall status of health and availability of other nutrients in the system. Effects of the micronutrients are more difficult to identify, partly because many of their actions occur at the cellular level, or even at the level of acting only on a certain component of the cell. Current levels of knowledge regarding adequacy and deficiency of many of the micronutrients are different from what they were ten years ago and no doubt, in time, our collective knowledge of the true range of functions of these substances will improve. For all of the essential microminerals, daily reference intakes (DRI) have been established and for most a tolerable upper limit (UL)[1].

Microminerals exist mainly in two forms, as charged ions, (bound to proteins), or in a complex within other molecules. They do not exist in the free ionic state. Each one has different properties that become critical in its functional role within the cell or other body tissues. Many enzymes require small amounts of one or more microminerals for full activity and minute quantities of microminerals affect the whole body through interactions with the enzymes, with hormones or the DNA in the nucleus of the cell. Seafood and fish are especially rich in most microminerals with the exception of manganese which is only available from plant sources of foods [1].

Iron

Iron has been recognised as an essential nutrient for more than a century. Despite the availability of iron-rich foods, iron deficiency anaemia remains the world's most common nutritional disorder. A healthy adult has between 2.4 g and 3.6 g total body iron in two pools, one being the functional iron found in the red blood cells and enzymes and the other being the ferritin found in the transport protein transferrin also in the blood. Iron is recycled by the body with about 90% being recovered from 'spent' red blood cells and brought back into the system. This still leaves 10% to be replenished on an average day [1]. A major function of iron is related to its ability to carry oxygen around the body bound to haemoglobin in the red blood cells. Iron is also necessary for the normal function of the immune system, the normal function of brain cells and the neurotransmitters in the nervous system. Deficiencies result in fatigue, lack of concentration and lowered immunity. Children who are deficient are compromised in their ability to learn, poor memory and retention of information and attention deficit [1].

There are two concerns with iron intake; one is that many people are still not getting enough, the other is that some people consuming large amounts of iron-fortified foods and supplements may be getting too much which could lead to haemochromatosis, an abnormal accumulation of iron in the liver and a propensity towards cardiac heart disease [1]. Iron in the diet is obtained in two different forms: one being haem iron found in large amounts in clams, oysters, fish and beef liver, the other being non-haem iron, good sources being baked beans, blackstrap molasses, lentils, wholegrain bread and fortified cereals. Non-haem iron is best consumed with some source of vitamin C for full absorption, such as tomatoes, orange juice or sweet peppers [1].

Zinc

Zinc is abundantly distributed throughout the body and is second only to iron in the amounts required. Zinc has only been known to be essential since the 1960s. Severe deficiencies have been found in Middle Eastern countries and amongst low-income families [1]. Vegetarians and those who are marginally nourished [1,15] are at risk for deficiency as the richest sources of this mineral are found in oysters, lean beef and turkey, although fortified cereals and wheat germ also provide significant amounts. Symptoms of deficiency include short stature, mild anaemia, decreased taste acuity, delayed wound healing, hair loss and skin lesions [1]. Phytates found in whole grains, and bran decreases the absorption of zinc, whilst the presence of protein increases it. Zinc is a component of more than 300 different enzymes that speed up reactions within the cell and participates especially in those reactions involving the degradation, or synthesis of proteins, lipids and carbohydrates. Zinc is also important for the stabilisation of protein structure and immune function [1]. Zinc deficiency has been linked to parasitic infestation [15] and the integrity of the gastrointestinal system [16].

Fluoride

Fluoride is a natural element found in soil and in all drinking water, although the fluoride content of both varies greatly around the world. Although not strictly considered an essential element, fluoride is important for the health of teeth and bones with approximately 2.5 mg fluoride contained in the average adult skeleton. The main function of fluoride is to harden the tooth enamel making it more resistant to dental caries it may also be an element in the hardening of bones. Fluoride, in addition, acts as an antibacterial agent in the mouth. Approximate recommended intakes for fluoride were only established as late as 1997, the standard recommendation being 1 ppm in community water supplies. Main sources of fluoride are drinking water and foods prepared with fluoridated water as well as seafood and saltwater fish and tea [1].

Because there is no known metabolic function for fluoride, true deficiency does not exist in functional terms; however, low levels will lead to an increase in dental caries. Mild fluorosis can occur if levels rise above 0.1 mg/kg body weight, resulting in discolouration of the teeth [1].

Copper

Copper is a normal constituent of blood and is an essential micronutrient. Concentrations in the body are highest in the liver, brain, heart and kidney as well as skeletal muscle. Copper is stored in the liver, and deficiency signs appear slowly over time. Copper is a component of many enzymes, and symptoms of copper deficiency are due to enzyme reaction failures. Signs of deficiency include anaemia, low white blood cell (neutrophil) counts and demineralisation of the skeleton as well as de-pigmentation of the skin (vitiligo) and hair. Food sources of copper include beef liver, pulses, blackstrap molasses, cashew nuts and sunflower seeds [1].

Iodine

Iodine is one of the ultra trace minerals and is present and required in only minute amounts. The main function of iodine is in the synthesis of two substances essential for the function of the thyroid gland: triiodothyronine (T_3) and thyroxine (T_4). Uptake of iodide by the thyroid gland is inhibited by goitrogens found in the cabbage family (cabbage and Brussel sprouts especially), turnips, peanuts, cassava sweet potatoes and soybeans, these are inactivated by cooking. Serious deficiency results in goitre, resulting in poor cognition and mental retardation, milder deficiency results in enlargement of the thyroid gland. In some countries, this condition is so common that it is felt by the indigenous population to be a normal feature. The richest food sources of iodine are seafood and saltwater fish as well as sea vegetables (nori and wakame), followed by freshwater fish and egg. Salt is commonly iodised in order to prevent deficiencies in vulnerable populations [1].

Selenium

Selenium has a very narrow range of beneficence; below which deficiency occurs and above which toxicity develops. Selenium is a component of Glutathione peroxidase (GSH-Px) an enzyme which acts together with antioxidant nutrients to scavenge free radicals from the system. Selenium is also found to be a component of several proteins formed in the body. Selenium deficiency is rare but has been found in China where the soil is particularly poor in this mineral. Symptoms of deficiency take some years to manifest themselves, resulting in Keshan disease, congestive cardiomyopathy caused by a combination of a dietary deficiency of selenium and the presence of a mutated strain of Coxsackievirus. It is named after Keshan County of Heilongjiang province, Northeast China, where symptoms were first noted. Additionally, smaller deficiencies over a period of time may contribute to carcinogenesis and the risk of cancer. The richest food sources of selenium are Brazil nuts, fish and seafood, molasses and sunflower seeds. Signs of toxicity include changes in skin and nails, tooth decay and non-specific gastrointestinal and neurological abnormalities [1].

Manganese

A healthy adult has approximately 10-20 mg of manganese in the body, mostly contained within the cells. This mineral is a component of some important enzymes and is essential for the active function of many more, most of which are associated with the formation of connective tissues and bones as well as carbohydrate and lipid metabolism. Symptoms of deficiency (first reported in 1972) include weight loss, dermatitis and, occasional nausea and vomiting, changes in hair colour and slow hair growth. The richest food sources of manganese are whole grains, legumes and nuts, whilst fruits and vegetables also contain moderate amounts [1].

Chromium

Although a biological role for chromium was discovered in 1954, it was not until 1977 that it was officially recognised as an essential mineral. Less than 2% of the chromium taken in from food sources is absorbed, although the presence of phytates in whole grains increases the absorption somewhat, as does iron deficiency. This fact, lead scientists to believe that the metabolism of chromium, was similar to that of iron. Strenuous exercise, trauma or higher sugar intakes increase the urinary excretion of chromium. The main function of chromium is to potentiate the effects of insulin, thereby increasing the efficiency of carbohydrate metabolism it appears in addition to having a beneficial effect on the lipid levels in the blood. Chromium deficiency results in insulin resistance and blood lipid abnormalities. The role of chromium as a glucose tolerance factor (GTF) is controversial, and supplements of chromium picolinate have resulted in adverse effects, primarily skin lesions. Good food sources of chromium include brewer's yeast, oysters, liver and potatoes and moderate amounts are also found in seafood and whole grains [1].

Cobalt

Cobalt in the body exists as a component of vitamin B12 which is essential for the maturation of red blood cells; it is also a component of one other essential enzyme which is involved in the conversion of nucleic acids and the formation of new cells [1].

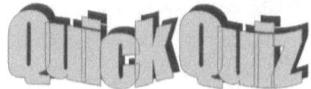

1. Which microminerals are involved in the health of bones and teeth?

    Answer: _____

    A. Cobalt and Chromium

    B. Iron and Zinc

    C. Fluoride

    D. Manganese

2. Which microminerals are involved in the health and function of red blood cells?

    Answer: _____

    A. Zinc and Copper

    B. Iron and Cobalt

    C. Fluoride and Chromium

    D. Manganese

3. Which microminerals are necessary for enzyme function?

   Answer: _____

   A. Zinc, Copper, Selenium and Manganese

   B. Fluoride, Copper, Zinc and Iodine

   C. Iron, Zinc, Cobalt and Fluoride

   D. Chromium, Cobalt and Iron

4. Which microminerals are required for the conversion of food to energy?

   Answer: _____

   A. Fluoride and Chromium

   B. Iron and Cobalt

   C. Iron and Zinc

   D. Chromium and Zinc

5. Which microminerals are essential for the function of the immune system?

   Answer: _____

   A. Fluoride and Cobalt

   B. Iron and Zinc

   C. Chromium and Manganese

   D. Selenium and Cobalt

Avoiding Mineral Imbalances

Consuming as wide a variety of food as possible will go a long way to avoiding deficiencies in minerals. Consider also the quality of food before the quantity. Although there are RDIs for the microminerals, they are often inexact, and the best way of ensuring neither too much nor too little is taken in, obtaining one's needs for food is a far better option than the hit and miss of various (and sometimes dubious) over the counter supplements of individual microminerals. Care is, however, needed with the microminerals to ensure not only adequate intake but adequate absorption and utilisation. Minerals are not so easy to destroy in cooking but many dissolve in water and steaming, grilling or stewing is the best way to cook food, if water must be used do not throw it away but use as a stock or soup base. In general, the following combinations of foods should be avoided:

Iodine rich foods:
Seafood, fish and sea vegetables such as nori and wakame as well as sushi
With: Raw cabbage, coleslaw and mixed lettuce and cabbage salad or raw peanuts

Zinc-rich foods:
Beef, turkey, oysters and seafood or wheat germ
With: High fibre cereals, wholegrain bread and breakfast cereals with added bran <u>Vegetarians would be well off adding a tablespoon of wheat germ to a fruit smoothie or vegetable soup</u>

The following food combinations go well together as some nutrients enhance the absorption of others:

Chromium rich foods:
Liver, potatoes, brewer's yeast and whole grains
With: High fibre foods such as cereals, muesli, lentils, beans and raw vegetables

Iron-rich foods:

Liver, seafood, fish, beans, lentils and wholegrain foods

With: foods rich in vitamin C such as tomatoes, peppers, broccoli and orange juice

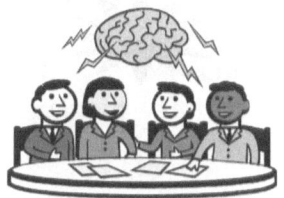

Learning Together

Learning Together

Activity 1: Allow yourselves 10 minutes for this activity

Looking at the foods that are rich in the essential minerals, you will notice that some are a good source of quite a number of these. The challenge in this exercise is for your group to try to find as few items as possible that will provide the full spread of minerals for:

a) A non-vegetarian
b) A vegetarian

You can decide between yourselves whether to include eggs and / or dairy products in the vegetarian choices. Do make this fun and don't make it a slog!

Write Your Notes Here

Activity 2: Allow yourselves 15 minutes for this activity

Looking at the foods you have chosen in the previous exercise, how do you think you can divide these foods between three meals for each group of people? What for instance would you put into:

a) Non-vegetarian breakfast
b) Non-vegetarian lunch
c) Non-vegetarian dinner
d) Vegetarian breakfast
e) Vegetarian lunch
f) Vegetarian dinner

Write Your Notes Here

Now you should take 5 minutes to discuss the results of your learning activities with your facilitator

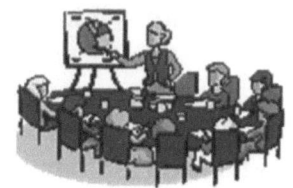

Discussion

Today's Topic for Discussion is THE SALT SCARE! TOO MUCH HYPE OR TOO LITTLE TOO LATE?

For thousands of years, we did without salt, it was a luxury that all but a few could afford, and there is no denying that it is not essential addition to our diet [6]. However, salt does enhance the flavour of particularly bland foods, hence its popularity in countries where few herbs and spices were traditionally used and its major role in the food manufacturing industry. It had become so popular that when a decision had to be made about finding something acceptable to which iodine could be added as a preventive of goitre, common table salt seemed a good choice at the time [1]. We now, however, consume daily on average far in excess of any possible need [1]. Hypertension (high blood pressure) is the major precursor to stroke and a major risk factor in cardiac heart failure which has increased not only in Westernised countries [17] but also in developing countries [18]. Diet and lifestyle have a substantial impact on the incidence of hypertension with obesity, lack of exercise, high sodium and low potassium intake being the main contributors [7]. Although the famous NHANES study conducted in the 1970s found a weak correlation between heart disease and salt intake, it was felt by the research group that it was still not enough evidence to warrant any particular dietary recommendation [19]. Many nutritional scientists and professionals involved in the public health arena feel that an effort to reduce the risks by curtailing sodium and increasing potassium would play a major role in enhancing both longevity and quality of health and life [6,8]. The American Heart Association nevertheless formally recommended a reduction in salt intake in 2006 [8].

Some questions to think about and to discuss as a group:

- Do you think that the fuss about salt is just that – a big fuss and that the individual should be left to look for their own information and decide for themselves whether to cut down on salt?
- Do you think that it is reasonable to give people both information about the risks pertaining to salt and reasonable alternatives and leave it to them?
- On the other hand, do you think that if there is adequate research about the dangers of too much salt, the government should be the ones to take charge of how much is sold and how much food manufacturers are allowed to use in the processing of foods?
- Do you think that the government and the food industry are taking too little responsibility for the problem and offering too few alternatives?
- It is very hard once one has got used to using salt to give this up – do you think that this should be approached in the same way as smoking and that people need help, support and some sodium free alternative flavourings on the national / government health system, or medical insurance system?
- Alternatively, you might feel that this is a two-way street and that the health authorities and the individual should both take steps to alleviate the problem of sodium intake.
- As a group overall, do you think that any action is needed and, if so, what would you advocate?

<u>You Might Like to Make Some Notes Here</u>

References

1. Anderson JJB. Minerals. In: Mahan LK, Stump SE (eds). Krause's Food Nutrition & Diet Therapy. 11th ed. Philadelphia: Saunders Elsevier, 2004.
2. Nordin BEC, Heaney RP. Calcium supplementation of the diet - justified by present evidence. British Medical Journal. 1990; 300:1056-60.
3. Altura BT, Brust M, Bloom S, Barbour RL, Stempak JG, Altura BM. Magnesium dietary intake modulates blood lipid levels and atherogenesis. Proceedings of the National Academy of Sciences. 1990; 87:1840-4.
4. Stipanuk MH. Metabolism of sulphur-containing amino acids. Annual Review of Nutrition. 1986; 6:179.
5. Nowak TJ, Handford AG. Pathophysiology: Concepts and Applications for Health Care Professionals. 3rd ed. New York: The McGraw - Hill Companies Inc.; 2004.
6. Frassetto L, Morris RC, Sellmeyer DE, Todd K, Sebastian A. Diet, evolution and ageing: The pathophysiological effects of the post-agricultural inversion of potassium-to-sodium and base-to-chloride ratios in the human diet. European Journal of Nutrition. 2001;40(5):200-13.
7. Geleijnse JM, Kok FJ, Grobbee DE. Impact of dietary and lifestyle factors in the prevalence of hypertension in Western populations. European Journal of Public Health. 2004;14(3):235-9.
8. Brookes L. New Dietary Advice, a New Government Program, A New Drug and a Truly Novel New BP Measurement Device. Medscape Cardiology. Volume 10, 2006:523827.
9. He FJ, MacGregor GA. Beneficial Effects of Potassium. British Medical Journal. 2001; 323:497-501.
10. Geleijnse JM, Grobee DE, Hofman A. Sodium and potassium intake and blood pressure change in childhood. British Medical Journal. 1990; 300:899-902.
11. Hughes J, Norman R. Diet and Calcium Stones. Canadian Medical Association Journal. 1992; 146:137-43.

12. Franco OH, Bonneaux L, deLaet C, Peeters A, Steyerberg EW, Machenbach JP. The Polymeal: a more natural, safer and probably tastier (than the polypill) strategy to reduce cardiovascular disease by more than 75%. British Medical Journal. 2004; 329:1447-50.

13. He FJ, Nowson CA, MacGregor GA. Fruit and vegetable consumption and stroke: meta-analysis of cohort studies. The Lancet. 2006; 367:320-6.

14. Food, Nutrition and the Prevention of Cancer, a Global Perspective. Washington DC: World Cancer Research Fund / American Institute for Cancer Research, 1997.

15. Hughes S, Kelly P. Interactions of malnutrition and immune impairment, with specific reference to immunity against parasites. Parasite Immunology. 2006; 28:577-88.

16. Thurnham DI. Micronutrients and immune function: some recent developments. Journal of Clinical Pathology. 1997; 50:887-91.

17. Kannel WB. Incidence and Epidemiology of Heart Failure. Heart Failure Reviews. 2000; 5:167-73.

18. Reddy KS, Yusuf S. Emerging Epidemic of Cardiovascular Disease in Developing Countries. Circulation. 1998; 97:596-601.

19. Alderman MH, Cohen H, Madhavan S. Dietary sodium and mortality: the National Health and Nutrition Examination Survey (NHANES I). The Lancet. 1998; 351:781-5.

LEARNING SESSION SEVEN: FIBRE AND PHYTONUTRIENTS

Introduction

Apart from the vitamins and minerals, two other frequently forgotten items of nutrition are fibre and the phytonutrients. Fibre comes in insoluble and soluble forms and constitutes a part of unprocessed foods of vegetable origin. We took a brief look at fibre as a component of carbohydrates, and in this session, we take a more in-depth view of both the various components of fibre and their role in health. We discuss how to avoid the problems that occur when not enough of this substance is taken in and what are the best forms to take in fibre.

In addition, we discover the often-overlooked phytonutrients. Substances of value that are often found in foods, herbs, spices and cooking ingredients are the phytonutrients. In this session, we look at some of these that clearly enhance our health and well-being, among them, are the microflora, which has a connection to fibre and to intestinal health. The advantages and possible considerations of phytoestrogens, garlic, turmeric and green tea will also be discussed.

We often miss out on the benefits of phytonutrients due to the way in which we prepare food and cultural preferences for a particular way of cooking. We look at traditional and more novel ways in which the benefits of these substances can be obtained and how we can incorporate them into our diet.

In the second part of our session we come to our learning together sessions where we lighten up our time together with some group endeavours and then on to our discussion for the day, 'gut feelings'; which is all about the bifidobacteria drinks on the market: are these a great idea or a bit of an expensive walk down the garden path? We take an in-depth look at the actual ingredients, the costs involved and the cost to benefit ratio and ask can we afford to do without these? Or is there another way of meeting our needs? We ask a few thought-provoking questions!

Fibre and its Role in Health

The definition of dietary fibre has broadened in the last few years as has our understanding of the mechanism by which foods and food components affect the human physiology. The American Association of Cereal Chemists definition of dietary fibre is: 'the edible parts of plants or analogous carbohydrates that are resistant to digestion and absorption in the human small intestine with complete or partial fermentation in the large intestine. Dietary fibre includes polysaccharides, oligosaccharides, lignin and associated plant substances. Dietary fibres promote beneficial physiological effects, including regulation of peristalsis, and possibly plays a beneficial role in blood cholesterol and blood glucose regulation [1].

We took a brief look at non-starch polysaccharides (NSP), commonly known as dietary fibre, in learning session two. NSP substances form the main constituent of what we have come to know as 'dietary fibre' however on a broader level we also now look at the oligosaccharides, gums, pectins and lignins that have fibre-like tendencies. Such substances are also precursors of the intestinal bacteria that are equally necessary to our health [2]. NSP is found only in foods of vegetable origin and mainly in those foods that have undergone little or no processing. The NSP component of foods is divided into two distinct types: homopolymers (insoluble less-fermentable fibre) and heteropolymers (soluble and more fermentable fibre) [3]. Homopolymers are the cellulose, fibrous walls of plants. They are rigid, less soluble and less fermentable than heteropolymers and are mainly contained in the structural parts of plants. Cellulose is the most abundant organic compound in the world constituting 50% or more of all the carbon in vegetation. It is found in the bran of grains as well as carrots, broccoli, celery and other vegetables [3].

Heteropolymers are formed from the internal cellular matrix of the plants. They are a modified form of cellulose that is less rigid, more fermentable and more soluble. These substances are hemicellulose structures and gums which have varying degrees of solubility. They include lignin and pectin, which are gel-forming fibres that are highly soluble [3]. Lignin has some antioxidant properties, and flaxseed lignin has phytoestrogenic properties and is currently under investigation for its possible role in the prevention of certain cancers and osteoporosis [3].

Insoluble Fibre			Soluble Fibre	
Cellulose	Hemicellulose	Lignin	Gums	Pectin
Whole Wheat	Whole Grains	Carrots	Oats	Apples
Bran	Bran	Turnips	Legumes	Citrus fruits
Vegetables		Potatoes	Barley	Strawberries
		Wheat	Guar gum	Carrots
		Seeds		
		Berries		

Research has shown that high intakes of dietary fibre confer a protective effect against carcinogenesis, leading to cancer of the colon, by binding with bile acids in the digestive tract and by a direct effect on the intestinal mucosa, also by indirect effect on the metabolism of carcinogens [4]. The strength of protection varies with the type of fibre, whilst increases in cellulose and hemicellulose (less fermentable) cereal fibre appear to confer the greatest protection against carcinogenesis. Fermentable soluble fibre appears to slow the absorption of sugars, thus decreasing the risks of blood glucose disorders [4]. Any increase in all types of fibre appears nevertheless to confer some benefit and studies reveal that colorectal cancer incidences are inversely related to the number of portions of fruits and vegetables consumed by an individual [5].

The risk of CHD is also decreased by the use of whole grain cereals and appears to be related to the intake of bran which reduces the amount of saturated fats absorbed, and researchers suggested that the intake of whole grain cereals be increased for persons predisposed to CHD [6]. This is borne out by a study that looked at two low-fat diets, one which incorporated low-fat meats and dairy products and the other which was identical in calorific value and nutrients but was plant-based. The plant-based diet considerably lowered total cholesterol and LDL levels far more effectively than the traditional low-fat diet normally prescribed for this problem [7].

Fructooligosaccharides

The two most common fructooligosaccharides (FOS) are inulin and the fructans. These are composed of fructose polymers often linked with an initial glucose molecule [3]. FOS is naturally poorly digested in the small intestine and only contributes approximately 1 calorie/gram to the starch intake in our diet[2,3]. Due to the fructose content, these have a clean, sweet taste, and are half as sweet as sugar. As such they may be useful as a natural alternative to sugar. FOS is found in more than 36,000 plant species, and diets that contain more fruits and vegetables are naturally higher in these compounds [3]. Major dietary sources include [3]:

- Wheat, barley and rye
- Onions and Garlic
- Bananas
- Chicory
- Asparagus
- Jerusalem artichokes
- Tomatoes

FOS reach the colon intact where it has its most important physiological effect, that of promoting the growth of beneficial colonic bacteria (microflora / probiotics)[3]. Research has shown that the higher the intake of FOS the higher the intestinal bacteria counts [8]. The FOS is hydrolysed by the intestinal bacteria into short-chain volatile acids and gases, which can result in bloating if a lot is taken in at once. Bloating, and bowel noises are, however, often seen at the beginning of the intake and at lower doses; when the dose is gradually increased these symptoms appear to lessen and go away completely in time [8]. Commercially, FOS are known as prebiotics and are often added to dairy products and yoghurt as well as some breakfast cereals [3].

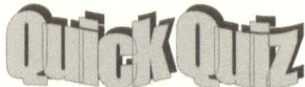

Using a different coloured pen or pencil for each food, match up the foods below to the type or types of fibre:

<u>Example</u>

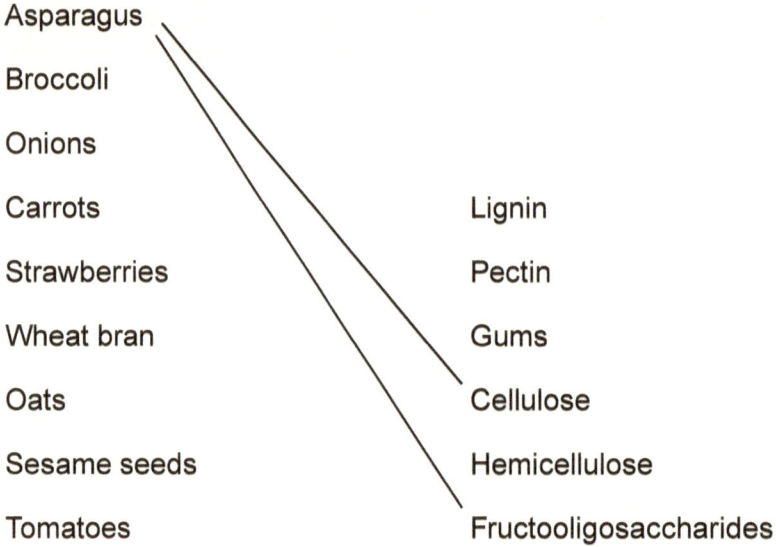

Asparagus

Broccoli

Onions

Carrots   Lignin

Strawberries   Pectin

Wheat bran   Gums

Oats   Cellulose

Sesame seeds   Hemicellulose

Tomatoes   Fructooligosaccharides

Celery

Whole grain rye bread

Apples

Turnips

Haricot beans

Phytonutrients: A Few Special Substances

Phytonutrients are not officially recognised as essential nutrients, but evidence to date suggests that these substances can enhance health. Bioflavonoids and FOS are technically phytonutrients, as these have already been discussed we will look at a few more that are commonly used and under increasing scientific scrutiny for possible benefits.

Microflora / The Probiotics

These substances are not really part of the plant matter that we normally associate with phytonutrients, but they are worth discussing in light of the fact that they are so often added to, or cultured within, commonly consumed food products. At birth, the intestinal tract is essentially sterile, but as soon as the infant begins to take in its mother's milk, micro-organisms develop with the aid of the FOS contained in the milk. Predominantly, the lactobacillus organisms flourish in the large intestine, followed by the formation of Escherichia coli once solid food begins to be taken. Generally the stomach and upper intestine remain almost bacteria free, but in the colon, hundreds of species of intestinal flora develop and flourish, lactobacilli continues to develop in people who consume a mixed diet [9].

Colonic bacteria fall into two groups: those that are putrefactive toxic acid producing substances (TAPS) and fermentative lactic acid producing substances (LAPS). It is the latter (LAPS) which plays a beneficial role in health and aid in the digestion of residual starches that have not been digested in the small intestine; during this process, some vitamin K and vitamin B12 is formed. In addition, these bacteria break down resistant starch and, in the process, dietary fibre is converted to short chain fatty acids that enhance the absorption of water and sodium and provides fuel for the cells of the intestine itself [9]. Intestinal disturbances and illnesses such as diarrhoea, irritable bowel syndrome, Crohn's disease and the use of antibiotics tend to disturb the balance of intestinal flora. In such cases and where dietary fibre intake is low, additional beneficial flora is required as are the FOS which help to regenerate a positive balance. Lactobacilli these are generally found in fermented dairy products such as yoghurt, fromage frais and cottage cheese. Supplements of multiple beneficial bacteria are also available.

Generally, foods which tend to either slow bowel transit time, or enhance colonic putrefaction also have a propensity to initiate the formation of TAPS. Examples of such foods are [4]:

- Beef
- Other fatty meats and cheeses
- Refined starches

Foods which tend to speed up bowel transit time, especially those rich in FOS tend to ferment. They also have the propensity to initiate and maintain the formation of LAPS such as [2,4]:

- Vegetables
- Fruits
- Whole grain cereals

Phytoestrogens

Phytoestrogens are plant chemicals, some of which structurally resemble endogenous oestrogens of humans and animals, and recent research suggests they may also function as oestrogen agonists or antagonists when eaten by humans. Although humans have used phytoestrogens medicinally for thousands of years, only in the last 25 years or so have researchers begun to look beyond the folk remedies to investigate phytoestrogens' possible roles in modern health care [10]. Phytoestrogens are those substances found in foods that mimic oestrogen activity in the body but to a relatively small extent. What is special about these substances is that they take up the places in the human cell that might otherwise be taken up by oestrogen-like damaging substances, or re-cycled used oestrogen transported from the intestines.

The most researched and, possibly the most useful, is genistein, a major isoflavone (a type of flavonoid) found in soy products [11]. Genistein has been shown to improve cardiovascular health and moderately enhance bone density in post-menopausal women in some studies [11]. Research shows that genistein has a beneficial effect on low-density lipoproteins, binding with these substances, preventing them from being oxidised thus preventing damage to the walls of the arteries which accounts, in part, for the benefits to the cardiovascular system [12,13]. In addition, the anti-angiogenic effects of genistein may also prevent the vascularisation of new tumours, thus preventing new tumour growth and cancers [13].

There have, however, been some concerns about the long-term use of a synthetically formulated supplement of genistein (ipriflavone), but no ill effects were found with short-term use of this supplement [11]. There has been no evidence found of ill-effects of long-term use of dietary genistein from the consumption of soy-based food products; however, these are culturally more acceptable in Chinese and Japanese populations. Recently, however, the world-wide availability of miso soup, tofu, soy milk and yoghurt have become more common and Westernised uses for soy has emerged with products such as tofu ice cream and soy-based 'pouring cream'.

Garlic

Garlic has been used in foods, as a preservative and as a folk remedy since recorded history began, at least in Europe, however, claims for its health benefits have only in recent years been scientifically evaluated. Fungal infections have become an important aspect of modern infectious disease practice. The prominence of fungi as pathogens may be due to the longer survival of immune compromised patients, the recent development and usage of broader-spectrum antibiotics, or the wider use of immunosuppressive and cancer chemotherapeutic agents. Garlic was used experimentally in 25 mg doses and, after 30 and 60 minutes, the antifungal residues were detected in the bloodstream;

however, this was short lived [14]. Scientists are now investigating whether the active ingredient in garlic, allicin, can be given in larger doses by injection for fungal infection.

Hypertension and high cholesterol and blood lipid levels are another chronic problem in health care; however, scientists have long wondered how come Mediterranean populations appear to have lower levels of blood lipids, despite the consumption of reasonable quantities of dairy products. The consumption of garlic may have something to do with this as research has found that raw crushed garlic has the effect of lowering blood pressure and blood lipid levels [15].

Helicobacter pylorus is a bacterium that is endemic in some populations, particularly in Africa. It is the cause of chronic gastritis and duodenal ulcers, problems that appear to be diminished in countries where garlic is eaten frequently as a part of the normal culinary culture. Laboratory research has found that garlic has the ability to destroy the Helicobacter pylorus bacterium and suggests that there is a future potential for its clinical use [16].

The main downside to garlic is the smell and the fact that its culinary acceptability is still very much connected to the Mediterranean peoples and their style of cuisine. Globalisation, migration and the increasing number of holidaymakers to the Mediterranean is slowly making garlic more culturally acceptable, and the odour of raw garlic can be offset with parsley and mint.

Turmeric

Turmeric is the common name for the 'Curcuma longa', also known as Indian saffron and is, in fact, a member of the ginger family of herbs. Turmeric is cultivated extensively in India, China and the Indonesian countries. The active ingredient is curcumin which has had traditional use as an antioxidant, anticarcinogenic, anti-inflammatory, and an antimicrobial [17]. It is the latter that has resulted in its wide use in cooking; as the main spice used in curries as in tropical climates, it was found to prevent food from microbial spoilage. Although the antioxidant and anti-inflammatory actions are possibly the most scientifically substantiated [18], the anticarcinogenic properties have been verified to date in both laboratory and animal studies. In humans, there has been found to be no toxic effect with a high dose intake of turmeric, and it now remains to be seen as to whether human trials will result in the use of this substance as a standard cancer preventative [19]. Unlike other spices, turmeric is relatively mild and well tolerated in cooking as well as being a useful and less expensive substitute for saffron as a food colouring and flavouring for rice. This along with its possible health benefits might aid in its more widespread Western use in the future.

Green Tea

Green tea has recently become a popular alternative to more traditionally drunk beverages such as black tea and coffee. Health claims have been made about its ability to provide a significant energy boost without the caffeine associated nervousness which accompanies strong tea and coffee. In addition, green tea appears to be tolerated well by those who find that black tea and coffee aggravates gastrointestinal problems. The main active ingredients in green tea are tannin and polyphenols. Tannin is an astringent that has been accredited with antioxidant and antimicrobial action [18]. An antioxidant-rich polyphenolic compound has been isolated from green tea and shown to have both anti-inflammatory and anticarcinogenic properties in experimental animals [20]. Taken together, a number of studies suggest that the phenols in green tea might be useful in the prevention and treatment of early onset arthritis [20].

A further possible medical use for green tea has also been found in the treatment of skin toxicity induced by radiotherapy. Skin toxicity causes skin disintegration and inflammation, decreasing the quality of life for cancer treatment patients and compromising further treatment. Topical application of both black and green tea reduced the inflammation of the skin lesions, but green tea was slightly more active and worked better in patients treated by abdominal radiation and those who had also been treated with chemotherapy [21]. Sepsis is another medical problem with a high mortality rate that has been found to respond favourably to regular consumption of green tea. It is thought that the polyphenols in green tea act as a mediator of the bacteria that cause sepsis and its resultant inflammation [22]. Although there is no research study to date, the soothing effects of green tea might be due to the anti-inflammatory action on the gastrointestinal lining which might account for its tolerability in those suffering from gastritis, duodenal or peptic ulcers and inflammatory bowel problems.

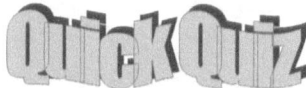

Using a different coloured pen or pencil for each food or beverage, match up the foods and drinks below on the left to the beneficial ingredients in the list on the right:

Vegetables

Goats milk yoghurt

Black tea   Curcumin

Garlic   Lactobacilli

Whole grain maize meal   Genistein

Curry powder   LAPS

Fruits   Allicin

Fromage frais   Phenols

Green tea

Soya yoghurt

Turmeric

Tofu

Balancing the Vegetable and Animal Foods in our Diet

In session ten, we will come to the whole issue of how to balance our individual food plans, however, at this point we will pause to take in an overview of what we require as individuals and which nutrients are available from where. In all, there is a broad spectrum of necessary nutrients as well as fibre, FOS, and other beneficial phytonutrients to be considered, which are available from a wide variety of sources, both animal and vegetable. Research has shown that the more vegetarian your diet looks, the more likely you are to be well nourished and the more nutritional protection from a disease you are probably afforded [23]. Choices as to how much or which foods of animal or vegetable origin one is prepared to eat may be made from cultural, religious, financial, ecological, practical or economic perspectives. Making an informed choice, however, requires that one has a reasonable amount of unbiased and factual information at hand to make the best decisions possible under the circumstances and without compromising one's freedom of belief.

We are going to look at which nutrients we can get from vegetable sources, which might be a little difficult and require some 'manoeuvring' in our dietary programme and which we can practicably only get from animal sources.

Obtainable from Vegetable Sources

Nutrients	Foods
Beta Carotene (which can be converted to Vitamin A)	Orange, yellow fruits and vegetables and dark green leafy vegetables
Vitamin E	Avocado pears, whole grains, nuts
Vitamin K	Dark green leafy vegetables
Thiamin, Riboflavin, Niacin, Pantothenic Acid	Whole grains, mushrooms, pulses, nuts

Vitamin C	Citrus fruits, berries, peppers, tomatoes
Calcium	Dark green leafy vegetables, soy beans
Phosphorous, Magnesium	Nuts, seeds, legumes
Sulphur	Soy beans, garlic
Sodium	Found in small amounts in most foods
Chloride	Green vegetables
Potassium	Fruits, vegetables, nuts
Iron	Beans, molasses, whole grains
Fluoride	Drinking water, tea
Copper	Beans, molasses, nuts and seeds
Selenium	Brazil nuts, molasses, sunflower seeds
Manganese	Whole grains, pulses, nuts
Chromium	Whole grains, potatoes, yeast
Soluble and insoluble fibre	Found in all foods of vegetable origin

Difficult to Obtain from Vegetable Sources

Nutrients	Foods
Vitamin D	Fish and fish liver oils, eggs
	An alternative source would be exposure to sunlight
Biotin, Zinc	Beef, pork, turkey, fish
	An alternative source would be cereals with added biotin and zinc
Iodine	Fish, seafood

Alternative sources would be sea vegetables and added iodised table salt

Can Only be Obtained from Foods of Animal Origin

Nutrients	Foods
B12	Meats, fish, eggs, yoghurt from sheep, goat's or cow's milk

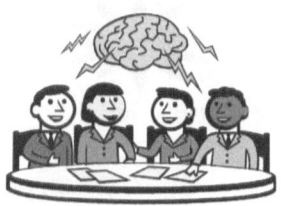

Learning Together
Learning Together

Activity 1: Allow yourselves 10 minutes for this activity

As a group, take one day in the week and list all the foods you have eaten between you on that day. Now look at this list and ask yourselves the following questions:

- Did you (as a group) miss out on any of the nutrients that you should have had?
- In general, what was the ratio of foods from vegetable to animal origin you consumed?

Write Your Notes Here

Activity 2: Allow yourselves 15 minutes for this activity

- Can you see where you might be able to shift the diet more towards foods of vegetable intake and still obtain a good supply of all the nutrients you need?
- Where do you think you may not be able to do this? Which nutrients would you not be able to obtain enough of if you ate a totally vegetarian diet?
- Take a look at your list and try to pick out the food items on it that would give the maximum intake of foods from a vegetable origin and still have all the nutrients one needs that everyone in your group would be happy to eat – or at least try to eat. (This might be challenging and do not be disappointed if you cannot please everyone!)

Write Your Notes Here

Now you should take 5 minutes to discuss the results of your activities with your facilitator.

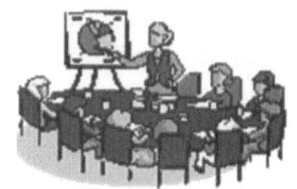

Discussion

Today's Topic for Discussion is GUT FEELINGS!

Lactose intolerance is more common than previously thought and a deficiency of lactase, the enzyme that digests lactose in milk, generally dies off around the time of weaning. It is now thought that this is, in fact, the norm with only about 15% of the Northern European population having a genetic anomaly that began about 10,000 years ago with the introduction of domesticated cattle and dairying in the Northern Hemisphere. This allowed the continuation of the lactase enzyme among Northern Europeans, but Native Americans, Asians and Africans tolerate milk poorly, hence traditionally amongst these cultures, milk which has a low lactose content (goats or sheep milk) has been favoured and has usually been fermented before drinking if it was consumed at all. This process used up the lactose and broke down some of the peptide bonds making the end-product easier to digest. Symptoms of lactose intolerance are abdominal bloating and gastrointestinal discomfort, often with pain and cramping as well as the formation of gas and, in severe cases, diarrhoea may occur [24]. Sugar is another product that ferments in the gastrointestinal system, also causing bloating and drawing water into the bowel. In excess, it counteracts the thiamine in the diet [3].

There is an awful lot of advertising lately about bifidobacteria and their benefits, much of it based on research. We do need some form of lactobacilli in our system, however, in one 45-minute slot on a popular radio station the author counted three adverts for a single yoghurt drink, purported to speed up gastrointestinal transit time and cut down bloating and intestinal discomfort. A children's version has also come on to the market recently. The product is sold in fruit flavoured 150 ml convenience sachets as a partly fermented thick sweet drink type of product. The cost of this product is R 1.67 [1]

The ingredients of this product are:

Skimmed milk	Fruit flavours
Cream	Colourings
Yoghurt Cultures	Stabilisers
Dextrose (sugar)	Preservatives
Corn syrup (sugar)	

A similar product making similar claims had the following ingredients:

Whole milk	Sugar
Skimmed milk concentrates	Glucose-fructose syrup
Cream	Stabilisers
Yoghurt cultures (Bifidus ActiRegularis)	Flavouring
Fruit	Acidity regulators

This product was fermented into a thick, smooth yoghurt(175 ml). The cost was R.14.50 [2] for 4 portions, i.e. R3.63 per portion per day.

A 1 Litre carton of plain yoghurt was found to contain:

Low-fat milk
Lactobacillus Acidophilus and Lactobacillus Bifidus –cultures
Stabiliser
The cost was R.19.50 15 for 6 x 167 ml portions, i.e. R3.25 per portion per day.

Some questions to think about and to discuss as a group:

- On a scale of 1 (not worth it) to 10 (very necessary and good value) how would you rate the above three products as far as usefulness, good health and economy are concerned?

---

[1]   US $ 0.14 c; UK £ 0.12 p
[2]   US $ 1.20 & 0.30 c UK £ 1.07 & 0.27 p and US $ 1.63 & 0.27 UK £ 1.44 & 0.24

- Do you think that some of these products and similar items have been a little 'hyped' by the media or would you say rather that the adverts are a form of public information?
- Overall do you think that we should be relying on commercial products to provide the necessary lactobacilli over a long period of time or do you think that it would be better to adjust the diet so that our bodies produce these necessary organisms internally?
- How practical do you think the above (3rd) solution might be?

<u>You Might Like to Make Some Notes Here</u>

References

1. The definition of dietary fibre. Cereal Foods World. 2001;46(112-126).
2. McCleary BV. Dietary fibre analysis. Proceedings of the Nutrition Society. 2003; 62:3-9.
3. Ettinger S. Macronutrients: Carbohydrates, Proteins and Lipids. In: Mahan LK, Escott-Stump S (eds). Krause's Food Nutrition & Diet Therapy. 11th ed. Philadelphia: Saunders Elsevier, 2004.
4. Reddy BS. Dietary fibre and colon cancer. Canadian Medical Association Journal. 1980; 123:850-6.
5. Joffe M, Robertson A. The potential contribution of increased vegetable and fruit consumption to health gain in the European Union. Public Health Nutrition. 2001;4(4):893-901.
6. Jensen MK, Koh-Bannergee P, Hu FB, et al. Intakes of whole grains, bran, and germ and the risk of coronary heart disease in men. The American Journal of Clinical Nutrition. 2004(80):1492-9.
7. Gardner CD, Coulston A, Chatterjee L, Rigby A, Spiller G, Farquhar JW. The Effect of a Plant Based Diet on Plasma Lipids in Hypercholesterolemic Adults. Annals of Internal Medicine. 2005; 145:725-33.
8. Bouhnik Y, Raskine L, Simoneau G, Paineau D, Bornet F. The capacity of short-chain fructo-oligosaccharides to stimulate faecal bifidobacteria: a dose-response relationship study in healthy humans. Nutrition Journal. Volume 5, 2006.
9. Beyer PL. Digestion, Absorption, Transport and Excretion of Nutrients. In: Mahan LK, Escott-Stump S (eds). Krause's Food, Nutrition & Diet Therapy. 11th ed. Philadelphia: Saunders Elsevier, 2004.
10. Barrett J. Phytoestrogens: Friends or Foes? Environmental Health Perspectives. 1996; 106:478-82.
11. Soung DY, Patade A, Kalil DA, et al. Soy protein supplementation does not cause lymphocytopenia in postmenopausal women. Nutrition Journal. Volume 5, 2006.

12. Tikkanen MJ, Wahalla K, Ojala S, Vihma V, Alderkreutz H. Effect of soybean isoflavone intake on low-density lipoprotein oxidation resistance. Proceedings of the National Academy of Sciences. 1998; 95:3106-10.

13. Fotsis T, Pepper M, Adlercreutz H, et al. Genistein, a dietary-derived inhibitor of in vitro angiogenesis. Proceedings of the National Academy of Sciences. 1993; 90:2690-4.

14. Carporaso N, Smith SM, Eng RHK. Antifungal Activity in Human Urine and Serum After Ingestion of Garlic. Antimicrobial Agents and Chemotherapy. 1983;23(5):700-2.

15. Jabbari A, Argani H, Ghorbanihaghjo A, Mahdavi R. Lipids in health and Disease. Volume 4, 2005.

16. O'Gara EA, Hill DJ, Maslin DJ. Activities of Garlic Oil, Garlic Powder and their Diallyl Constituents against Heliobacter pylori. Applied and Environmental Microbiology. 2000;66(5):2269-73.

17. Murray MT, Bongiorno PB. Curcuma longa (Turmeric). In: Pizzorno JE, Murray MT (eds). Textbook of Natural Medicine. Volume 1. St. Louis: Churchill Livingstone Elsevier, 2006.

18. Cowan MM. Plant Products as Antimicrobial Agents. Clinical Microbiology Reviews. 1999;12(4):564-82.

19. Lao CD, IV MTR, Normolle D, et al. Dose escalation of a curcuminoid formulation. BMC Complementary and Alternative Medicine. Volume 6, 2006.

20. Haqqi TM, Anthony DD, Gupta S, et al. Prevention of collagen-induced arthritis in mice by a polyphenolic fraction from green tea. Proceedings of the National Academy of Sciences. 1999; 96:4524-9.

21. Pajonk F, Riedisser A, Henker M, McBride WH, Fiebich B. The effects of tea extracts on pro-inflammatory signalling. BMC Medicine. Volume 4, 2006.

22. Chena X, Lia W, Wanga H. More tea for septic patients? - Green tea may reduce endotoxin-induced release of high mobility group box 1 (HMGB1) and other pro-inflammatory cytokines. Medical Hypotheses. 2006;66(3):660-3.

23. Food, Nutrition and the Prevention of Cancer, a Global Perspective. Washington DC: World Cancer Research Fund / American Institute for Cancer Research, 1997.

24. Beyer PL. Medical Nutrition Therapy for Lower Gastrointestinal Disorders. In: Mahan LK, Escott-Stump S (eds). Krause's Food, Nutrition & Diet Therapy. 11th ed. Philadelphia: Saunders Elsevier, 2004.

LEARNING SESSION EIGHT: THE ESSENTIAL ELEMENTS

Introduction

In this session we look at the three items we really and truly cannot live without and yet we do not think of them in traditional terms as essential nutrients, in fact, we do not often think of them at all! The essential elements of water, air and sunlight, without which there would be no life on the planet, including our own existence, is the focus of this learning session. Here we look at what we need in terms of the essential elements and how best to obtain them, how much we require for health and what is the best way of improving the quality of what we have.

Water is a bit controversial these days, it not only comes out of the tap (for most of us that are) but also in bottles of varying types and qualities which we might boil, filter, or add substances to. We look at our body's needs for water, the signs and symptoms of dehydration and how to avoid this problem. We also take a look at obtaining the best quality water that we can given our circumstances and the best ways to consume fluids.

We then go on to air, clean air and good quality air as well as the correct way to breathe. We look at what happens when we are only slightly short of oxygen and how to get a good supply under less than ideal circumstances. Finally, we look at the sunlight which we need, not only as a source of vitamin D but also in order to build an essential neurotransmitter, serotonin. We look at what happens when we have too little as well as too much and how to maintain a sensible balance.

Finally, we come to our learning together sessions where we engage in some interesting and fun group activities. We then move on to our discussion for this session – seeing the trees for more than the woods. For thousands of years, the trees gave us food and clean air until we discovered furniture, fuel and paper. Although we need land for agriculture, can we find a balance – what is in a tree for us? Can we turn things around even if it is only on a small scale for ourselves and our families? You might be surprised to find out what you can get out of a couple of patio pots!

Water and Hydration

Water is the largest single component of the body, and the volume, distribution and composition of the body fluids have profound effects on the function of the individual cells, tissues organs and the metabolic balance of the body as a whole. The cells of the muscles and viscera have the highest water content in the body and the calcified tissues of bones and teeth the least. Athletes, and those with a relatively high proportion of lean body mass have a higher water content than those less active and as one ages and the lean tissue mass depletes, the water content of the body also diminishes[1]. On average, a healthy man of average weight and fitness will have a total body water content of 60% and a healthy average woman a total body water content of 55%[2].

Of the total body water content, 2/3 will be intracellular fluid, that is the fluid inside the cells, and 1/3 extracellular fluid, that is the fluid outside of the cells. Much of this (80%) is the fluid surrounding the cells, commonly termed 'interstitial fluid' and 20% is plasma (the liquid portion of the blood)[2]. This is shown better in the chart below.

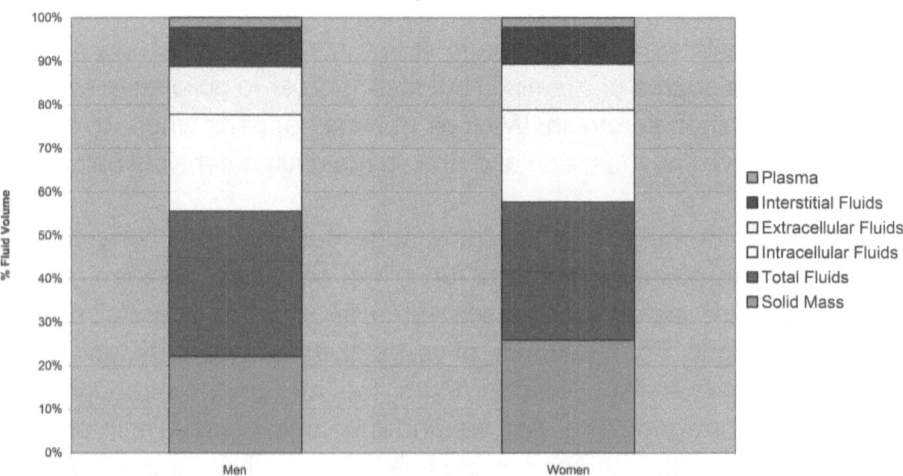

Total Body Water Ratios

© A. A. Morris-Paxton 2019

Water is the universal solvent and is vital for all the body's enzymatic and metabolic functions. The body has no ability to store water, and the water lost each day needs to be replenished. Water comes from only one of three sources, foods, fluid intake and water of metabolism, which is the water yielded from the chemical conversion of food to energy. The water of metabolism, accounts for between 200 ml and 300 ml of water per day, depending on the amount of food eaten and the efficiency of its conversion. The remainder needs to be taken in via the food and beverage content of the diet [1]. Total water gains need to meet the total water losses of approximately 2,500 ml per day. Approximately 1,600 ml is lost from kidneys and 100 ml in the faeces; another 600 ml is lost from skin and 300 ml from lungs [2].

Water Gains

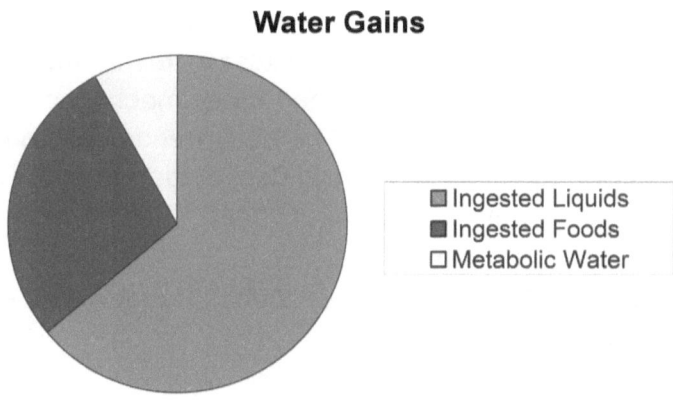

Water Losses

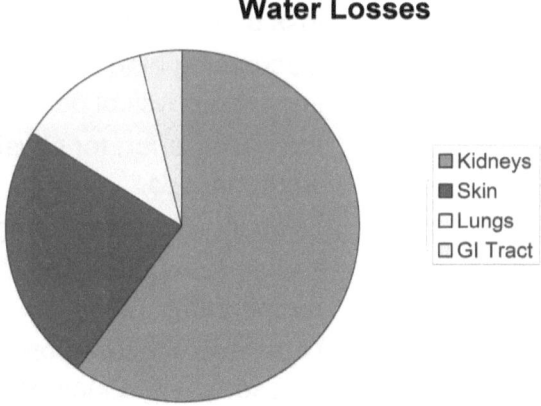

When the required amount of water taken in by ingestion and the water of metabolism equals the water lost then the body is said to be in *fluid balance*. However much can go wrong with this balance and keeping the balance constant requires that the water of metabolism is generated via the generation of energy and that enough fluid is taken in as well as the correct foods [2]. When a diet is rich in fresh fruits vegetables, cooked grains, pulses and fresh nuts which hold water, then less will have to be drunk. A fat rich and / or protein-rich diet, however, which contains few fruits and vegetables will not only yield less in fluids but may require more fluids to be digested, necessitating a greater fluid intake.

Dehydration occurs when water loss is greater than water intake, meaning that there is a decrease in the volume of water and an increase in osmolarity (the ability of the fluids to pass across the cell membranes) of the body. Water losses result first in fatigue followed by thirst generated by a feedback mechanism resulting from the increase in osmolarity. The body needs only to lose 2% of its mass due to fluid loss for mild dehydration to occur and the symptoms of dehydration to be experienced [2].

% of body weight lost through water losses	Symptoms of dehydration:
0-1%	Fatigue
2	Thirst, vague discomfort and loss of appetite
3	Decreasing blood volume and impaired physical performance
4	Increased effort for physical work, nausea
5	Difficulty in concentrating
6	Failure to regulate body temperature
8	Dizziness, laboured breathing on exertion and increased weakness

10	Muscle spasms, delirium and wakefulness
11	Circulatory collapse and kidney failure

Children and infants are at risk from mild dehydration with mild acute bouts of non-specific diarrhoea. Best treatment involves giving clear fluids such as cooled herbal teas (Rooibos / Redbush tea contains minerals and antioxidants) and diluted clear apple juice are good choices. Milk and dairy products should be stopped for at least 24 hours and the clear fluids given followed by the BRAT diet (bananas, rice cereal, applesauce and toast)[3]. Although the requirement for fluids is slightly less as one ages, there is a natural tendency for the sensation of thirst to diminish making older persons more vulnerable to dehydration. Dehydration has been responsible for about 10% of hospitalisation of the state dependent elderly in the US and may account for approximately 1-2% of all hospital admissions. Risk of dehydration increases with age, and it is more likely that risk is further increased with the onset of chronic illness, such as respiratory difficulties or diabetes [4]. Chronic mild dehydration that is not necessarily clinically detectable, but is due to long-term slightly inadequate fluid intake, is associated with constipation, an increased risk of kidney stones, decreased salivation and an increased risk of certain cancers as well as childhood obesity [1].

Increased fluid intake is also necessary with increased ambient temperature, sunbathing, exposure, exercise and increased perspiration due to strenuous exercise. Infection, illness, fever and stress will also increase the body's requirement for fluids, as will fasting, decreased appetite and long periods spent in dry air-conditioned surroundings [1].

Water balance, for practical purposes, is maintained by that which is ingested. Provided that five portions of fruits and vegetables are taken in, alongside other fresh foods which contain enough fluid for their own digestion, 1600 ml of water is needed as drinking water [2]. This applies to those of average weight, height and build and living in a temperate climate; however, there is a more exact way of calculating fluid needs [1] which we will go through in our 'learn together activity'.

Water can be obtained in several ways, some of which are a better source of fluids than others. In order of choice these are [1,3]:

Pure water (with no change in taste, smell or colour)
Rooibos (red bush) tea
Fruit or herbal infusions
Clear diluted apple juice
Low sodium clear vegetable broth
Diluted clear fruit juices
Decaffeinated black tea
Freshly squeezed juices
Soda water
Light, thin soups

Milk and caffeinated drinks do not count towards the overall fluid intake for rehydration purposes. Milk is very concentrated and, for infants, more of a food source; the lactose can aggravate intestinal problems and may increase diarrhoea [3]. Caffeinated drinks may exacerbate dehydration, as do alcoholic drinks [1]. Drinking water sources may need to be monitored, as research shows that both tap water and bottled waters contain varying amounts of minerals, especially calcium, magnesium and sodium. Magnesium and calcium, present in hard water, has been shown to decrease cardiac heart disease; however, soft water is high in sodium content and over time can increase the risk for this disease. Bottled water, if drunk on a continuous basis, may need compensating for in the rest of the food and fluid intake, especially if the sodium content is high [5]. Although filtering water for domestic use takes out some of the minerals, the chlorine used to decontaminate recycled water also leaves water exposed to further bacterial contamination. This needs to be refrigerated and drunk within a few hours of filtering. Filters need to be changed on a frequent basis. Reverse osmosis is the safest and most effective way of removing any chemicals or impurities from water, but reverse osmosis filters are expensive.

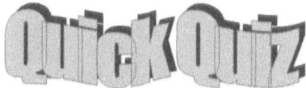

Look at the list of items below and decide which of these may be good, not great but passable and not very useful contributions to overall fluid requirements.

1. Circle the items you think are good sources of fluids in green

2. Circle the items you think are not very good but passable sources of fluids in yellow

3. Circle the items you think would not make a useful contribution to one's fluid intake in red

Cappuccino   V8 vegetable juice   Sparkling mineral water

Diluted clear red apple juice   Banana honey and yoghurt smoothie

Peppermint tea   Sloe gin and tonic water   Filtered tap water

Freshly squeezed carrot juice   Thick cream of chicken soup

Diluted cranberry juice   Tomato Cocktail   Beef tea

Hot chocolate with marshmallows and cream   Elderflower infusion

Air and the Oxygen We Need

Although we traditionally think of respiration as something we do with our lungs, in fact, it is something we do with our cells. Respiration is the process of gas exchange in our bodies, and it has three basic steps [2]:

1. Pulmonary ventilation, or breathing, is the inflow and outflow of air between the atmosphere and the alveoli (small sponge-like tissues) of the lungs [2].
2. External respiration is the exchange of gases (oxygen and carbon dioxide) between the alveoli and the red blood cells [2].
3. Internal respiration is the exchange of gases between the red blood cells in the capillaries and the tissue cells of the organs of the body. Without this oxygen, the individual cells cannot produce energy or carry out any other metabolic chemical reaction [2].

To a large extent, all of this goes on without our conscious knowledge or control; however, the whole process begins with the pulmonary ventilation – breathing, which has two stages to it, that of inspiration (inhalation or breathing in) and expiration (exhalation or breathing out). Just before inspiration, the air pressure inside the lungs is equal to the pressure of the air outside. For air to flow in, the pressure inside needs to drop which is accomplished by the diaphragm (the muscle at the base of the chest cavity) moving down to expand lung volume, allowing air to flow in. The oxygen then moves across the alveoli into the blood and cells, and the carbon dioxide is carried back to the lungs, through the alveoli and expired (breathed out). This is accomplished by the diaphragm moving up, contracting the lung capacity, creating a higher pressure inside than outside and the air flows out [2].

There are two preconditions to all of this happening with ease and for the body to obtain the right amount of oxygen for its needs. The first is that breathing is unobstructed, normal and without undue strain. The second is that the air we take in is clean, of good quality and has adequate oxygen content. The term for normal quiet breathing is *eupnoea* and which usually consists of a pattern of both shallow and deep breathing. Shallow breathing is known as *costal breathing* and consists of an upward and outward movement of the chest filling only the top ¼ to ½ of the lungs. A pattern of deep abdominal breathing where the diaphragm pulls down to its fullest extent, expanding the abdomen and filling the lungs is known as *diaphragmatic breathing* [2].

Bad breathing habits can be developed just as bad eating habits can be developed over time. Hyperventilation syndrome is a collection of problems caused by breathing pattern disorders. Some of these are due to an organic functional problem that requires medical diagnosis and correction; however, often acute hyperventilation can be due to nervous over-reaction to a stressful event, bronchial spasm, or an acute hypoglycaemic (low blood glucose) attack. A short-term problem can become a chronic long-term problem if not recognised and dealt with sufficiently. The good news is, however, that good breathing habits can be cultivated with correct breathing exercises, and a chronic shallow breather can learn to breathe deeply and evenly [6]. Physical therapy rehabilitation of breathing is summarised in the acronym [7] :

B   Breathing retraining
E   Esteem / self-image
T   Total body relaxation
T   Talk / breath control
E   Exercise prescription
R   Rest / sleep

Although there is virtually no more debate about whether or not our world has become polluted, there is a considerable amount of debate as to whether or not the pollution has reached high enough levels to cause adverse effects [8]. People are exposed to a variety of chemicals and possibly toxic substances in the food they eat, substances they come into contact with, the products they use and the air they breathe [9]. Chronic obstructive pulmonary disease (COPD) is not an organic or functional disease due to an internal fault, or invasion by bacteria or viruses; it is solely because of breathing in noxious fumes and chemicals, the main cause of which is smoking. Asthma too is on the increase and is aggravated by poor air quality and stressful life situations [10].

In the last decade, the burden of disease in developing countries due to the use of biomass fuels (predominantly wood but also coal and charcoal) has been found to be significant. In India alone approximately 400,000 – 550, 000 premature deaths might be attributed to the damage done by the consistent use of biomass fuels. Women at home with children are predominantly at risk. Using a disability-adjusted lost life year approach, the burden is estimated at 4-6 life years per person in India alone [11].

Aside from correct breathing and management of stress and respiratory disorders, there are two things we can do with respect to the quantity and quality of oxygen intake. One is to remove from our environment as many noxious substances as possible, and the other is to make small changes to our surroundings in order to improve our own personal 'airspace'.

Some ways we can remove noxious substances from our immediate environment include:

1. Giving up smoking (the author is not even pretending this is easy!). Research has shown that smoking cessation with group support is easier than if you try this alone and you are more likely to be successful if doing it together with others [12].
2. Eliminating the burning of fossil fuels, such as coal and wood where possible, as the smoke produces both carbon monoxide and carbon dioxide which are damaging to health in the long term [13]. Ventilate homes adequately and find other sources of warmth and cooking facilities such as electricity and piped gas.
3. Keeping homes well ventilated and free from damp as well as vacuuming regularly, or sweeping (with doors and windows open) will help to eliminate dust mites which can aggravate the airways of susceptible individuals [13].

4. Research has shown an increase in asthma, especially in children, is connected to road traffic pollution [14]. Don't go for your early morning run next to the traffic, instead drive to the nearest park and close the car windows if stuck in a jam.

Ways in which we can enhance our personal airspace quality include:

1. Getting out into the garden – a walk in a green and peaceful area during the day provides not only relaxation which in itself is an aid to better breathing[6], but also provides a better quality of air and oxygenation [15].
2. Plants and miniature trees in the office and home environment will aid in the absorption of carbon dioxide and the repletion of oxygen in the air [15], which is especially beneficial in a crowded environment such as an open plan office.
3. Conversely, remove plants from the bedroom at night as this is the time when carbon dioxide is given off and bring them back again in the morning.
4. Take time to breathe, especially if anticipating a stressful meeting or event, stand near an open window (preferably next to a garden or lawn) or go for a quick 'walk break' away from the traffic and take ten slow deep abdominal breaths. Deep breathing will aid relaxation and provide more oxygen to the brain which in turn is more likely to be both calming as well as promoting mental alertness [6].

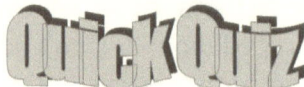

Look at the list of items below and decide which of these may be good, not great but passable and not very useful contributions to improving the quality of your personal 'airspace'.

1. Underline the items you think are good contributions in green

2. Underline the items you think are not very good but passable contributions in yellow

3. Underline the items you think would not make a useful contribution in red

a) Sitting near the window in a smoky nightclub

b) Opening the window nearest the garden in a stuffy office

c) Having a pot plant on or near your desk at work

d) Planting a tree in your garden outside the room your family uses the most

e) Deep breathing exercises at your office desk in the coffee break

f) Turning on the air conditioning when a meeting room starts filling up with people

g) Spending the lunch break relaxing with a book on the outside steps of an industrial plant

h) Going for an early morning run along the busy main road

i) Going outside for a walk in the park in the lunch break and doing some breathing exercises in the open air about halfway through

Sunlight, Good and Bad – Maintaining the Balance

The use of sunlight for health (heliotherapy) dates back to ancient Roman and Greek times [16] and has been a treatment option for practising naturopaths since the inception of naturopathic medicine [17,18]. However, modern health professionals have for some years been advocating a retreat from sunlight and the use of protecting skin creams even with minimum exposure [19]. Sunlight is a two-edged sword; whilst we need this essential element for life and health, we also have to be cautious about the possibilities and consequences of overexposure to the sun. Sunlight contains several forms of light rays the best known of which are the UV (Ultraviolet) rays, which are responsible for the production of two essential substances, vitamin D needed for bone health and strength of the skeletal system and Serotonin, a neurotransmitter needed for the correct functioning of the nervous system. Sunlight is, in addition, an antibacterial and often used for the treatment of skin disorders [19].

Vitamin D–deficiency rickets is a sunlight deficiency disease. The inability to appreciate the beneficial effect of sunlight on health had devastating consequences for both children and adults for more than 300 years. When it was finally realized that exposure to sunlight could prevent and treat rickets, the recommendation was made that all children be exposed to sensible sunlight in order to maximize bone health [20]. One hour of sunlight exposure can produce the equivalent of 10,000 IU of vitamin D without toxicity, as the process is self-limiting and only the amount of vitamin D that the body can utilise will be produced [21]. Vitamin D is especially important in the prevention of osteoporosis and the strengthening of bone. If maximum bone strength can be attained in the younger years, this serves to lessen the risk of osteoporosis later in life. The elderly and frail who do not go out into the sun are especially at risk of both fracture and the reduction of healing and prolongation of recovery from a fracture [22] [20].

The fortification of milk with vitamin D eradicated rickets as a major health problem, and, therefore, it was thought to have been conquered. Rickets has, however, made an unfortunate comeback. The major cause of rickets in the United States is a lack of appreciation that human milk contains very little if any vitamin D to satisfy the infant's requirement. African American women are often vitamin D deficient, and women who always wear sun protection and only take a prenatal multivitamin are also at high risk of vitamin D insufficiency. If they provide breast milk to their infant as the sole source of nutrition, the infant will become vitamin D deficient. If the infant is not exposed to sunlight or does not receive a vitamin D supplement, the infant will inevitably develop rickets. However, the skeletal manifestations of rickets represent only the tip of the vitamin D deficiency iceberg. Vitamin D deficiency in utero and during the first year of life has devastating consequences and may imprint on the child's life, resulting in chronic diseases that will shorten his or her lifespan. In utero, vitamin D deficiency results in reduced intrauterine long bone growth and slightly shorter gestation. This has been linked to increased risk of osteoporosis and fractures later in life. Children born and raised at latitudes below 35° for the first 10 years have a 50% reduced risk of developing multiple sclerosis later in life. Neonates who are vitamin D deficient during the first year of life are 2.4-fold more likely to develop type 1 diabetes compared with children who received 2,000 IU of vitamin D3 per day [20].

Seasonal Affective Disorder (SAD) is a type of depression that worsens in the winter months and is improved in the summer months with increasing exposure to sunlight. Full spectrum light therapy had been seen to be effective for this disorder as it increases the production of serotonin which, in turn, increases the production of melatonin, the neurotransmitter responsible for the regulation of sleeping and waking cycles and mood [23].

There is some controversy surrounding the risk of malignant melanoma (a form of skin cancer) and sunlight exposure [19,21]. The widespread concern about any direct sun exposure increasing the risk of the relatively benign and non-lethal squamous and basal cell cancers needs to be put into perspective. It is chronic excessive exposure to sunlight and sunburn during childhood that increases the risk of non-melanoma skin cancer. Melanoma, one of the most feared cancers because of its ability to rapidly metastasize before it is obvious to either the patient or physician, has been branded as a sun-induced skin cancer [20]. Most melanomas occur, however, on the least sun-exposed areas. Evidence from several studies has found that the non-exposed surfaces of the skin have a higher incidence of melanoma than the exposed surfaces and it has been reported that occupational exposure to sunlight decreases the risk of melanoma [20,21].

The 30-year campaign to recommend abstinence from sun exposure has not stemmed the increase in skin cancer incidence. It is curious that in the 1930s and 1940s when children were encouraged to be exposed to sunlight and artificial UV radiation to treat rickets, the incidence of skin cancer did not increase. The peak of skin cancers appeared however in the 1970s and, since then, the American Academy of Dermatologists has advised against any therapeutic use of sunlight and maintains that all vitamin D should be obtained from foods and supplements [16]. It is interesting to note that in Turkey, the estimated figures for skin cancers of all types are 5-7% of the total cancer burden; however, 6% of all children under three years suffer from vitamin D deficient rickets [16]. Although sunscreen use is generally advised when exposed to the sun, there is the risk of photo-instability of many of these commercial products, which may lead to a false sense of security at best and an increase in skin damage at worst [24]. Thus, there needs to be a re-evaluation of the beneficial effect of sensible exposure to sunlight as noted by the Australian College of Dermatologists and the Cancer Council Australia, which recommend a balance between avoiding an increased risk of skin cancer and achieving enough UV radiation to maintain adequate vitamin D levels [19,20].

Based on the current research available, it appears that potential benefits of sunlight outweigh the risks for short-term careful exposure [19]. The following guidelines might be useful:

- For infants, 20 minutes per day outdoor exposure to sunlight is adequate [16]
- 15 minutes up to one hour of sun exposure is safe and effective for adults, providing that after the first 15 minutes, a dermatological recommended protective lotion or cream should be applied.
- Frequent short-term exposure is better than single long periods of exposure, and exposure should be built up slowly, beginning with 10 minutes and increasing by 5 minutes every few days.
- Sunning should be avoided between 10.00 am and 3.00 pm

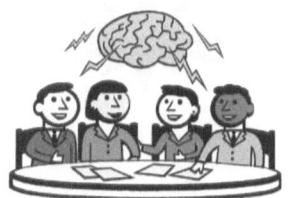

Learning Together

Learning Together

Activity 1: Allow yourselves 15 minutes for this activity

Hopefully, one member of your learning group will volunteer for this exercise, or choose one between you, to calculate their fluid requirements. Now follow the steps below:

1. Take your volunteer's approximate weight in Kg
2. For the first ten Kg allow   1,000 ml
3. For the second 10 Kg allow   500 ml
4. For persons under 50 years allow 20 ml per Kg for the rest of the weight in Kg   ?
5. For persons older than 50 years allow 15 ml per Kg for the rest of the weight in Kg   ?
    Sub Total   _____

6. If the person is consuming three meals and 200 ml two snacks per day (and therefore, taking in an average 2,500 Cal per day) deduct
7. For each approximate 500 Cal over this, deduct 50 ml another
    Sub Total   _____

8. For each approximate 500 Cal under the 50 ml average, add back to the subtotal above
    EVERYONE
9. For each portion of fruit and vegetables 50 ml consumed deduct

               TOTAL REQUIREMENTS   _____

Write Your Notes Here

Activity 2: Allow yourselves 10 minutes for this activity

a) As a group, look at each person's exposure to the sun this week, add this up in hours
b) Multiply by 4 to get the number of 15-minute sun time units.
c) Divide this figure again by the number of people in your group to obtain the average sun time units per person.

As 15 minutes sun exposure (1 sun time unit) gives 10 µg – 40 µg vitamin D (not an exact science), answer the following:

1. Did everyone get enough sunshine on average?
2. If not, what foods would you need to have eaten to make up for the lack of sunlight?

<u>Write Your Notes Here</u>

Now you should take 5 minutes to discuss the results of your activities with your facilitator.

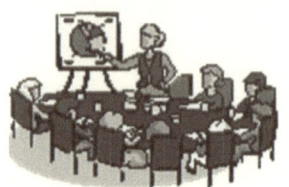

Discussion

Today's Topic for Discussion is: SEEING THE TREES FOR MORE THAN THE WOODS

In recent years, an increasing amount of research has linked changes in forest cover to several diseases, including some types of yellow fever and others, in particular, parasitic diseases, previously thought to be under control. The role that diminishing forest cover has in the global increase in infectious disease may in some scientist's views be its most direct impact on the health of humanity, albeit not the only impact. In the longer term the intentional deforestation in order to provide land for farming, housing and industry, as well as the increasing demand for wood products (furniture, timber for building and paper), involved losses of potential sources of medicines, as well as increasing air and water pollution. The most dangerous emissions are those of carbon dioxide and mercury gas into the air. In addition, the concomitant rise in global temperature is permitting certain types of malaria to flourish in areas where it has not existed before moving from tropical to what were once more temperate zones. Extremely worrying to scientists is the loss of the ecosystems that filter toxins from air and water supplies, as well as diluting the strength of the sun's UV rays, thus polluting two of our most basic nutrient resources and changing our exposure levels to the third. Forests purchased for watershed represent the cleanest and most effective use of forest land, as well as providing food sources for people in the form of fruits, nuts, seeds and mushrooms as well as for animal life [15].

Some questions to think about and discuss as a group:

- Given the fact that the following can be grown in a large pot, or in a trough over a fence or balcony rail:

© A. A. Morris-Paxton 2019

- Miniature plum tomatoes and cherry tomatoes
- Avocado pears
- Apricots
- Lemons, limes and tangerines (nartjies)
- Blackberries and raspberries
- Green beans and peas

How much of a contribution do you think you could make to your nutritional status, and air quality in the space that you currently have, be it a garden, patio or balcony?

- What else can you think of that you might do to contribute to:
  - Your own personal food supplies
  - Your quality of personal airspace
  - The amount of clean water you have, or the way in which you currently use water in your own home and garden or balcony?

- Do you think that the act of doing something rather than nothing to improve your nutrition and surroundings will at least make people feel less of a victim and more empowered about their ability to take control of their own situation?

You Might Like to Make Some Notes Here

References

1. Whitmire SJ. Water, Electrolytes and Acid-Base Balance. In: Mahan LK, Escott-Stump S (eds). Krause's Food Nutrition & Diet Therapy. 11th ed. Philadelphia: Saunders Elsevier, 2004.
2. Tortora GJ, Derrickson B. Principles of Anatomy and Physiology. 11 ed. Hoboken: John Wiley & Sons Inc.; 2006.
3. Smith LG. Teaching Treatment of Mild, Acute Diarrhoea and Secondary Dehydration to Homeless Parents. Public Health Reports. 1987;102(5):539-42.
4. Warren JL, Bacon E, Harris T, McBean AM, Foley DJ, Phillips C. The Burden and Outcomes Associated with Dehydration among US Elderly. American Journal of Public Health. 1994;84(8):1265-9.
5. Azoulay A, Garzon P, Eisenberg MJ. Comparison of the Mineral Content of Tap Water and Bottled Waters. Journal of General Internal Medicine. 2001; 16:168-75.
6. Chaitow L. Hyperventilation Syndrome / Breathing Pattern Disorders. In: Pizzorno JE, Murray MT (eds). Textbook of Natural Medicine. 3rd ed. Volume 1. St. Louis: Churchill Livingstone Elsevier, 2006.
7. Bradley D. Physiotherapy breathing rehabilitation strategies. In: Chaitow L, Bradley D, Gilbert C (eds). Multidisciplinary approaches to breathing pattern disorders. Edinburgh: Churchill Livingstone, 2002.
8. Crinnion WJ. Environmental Medicine. In: Pizzorno JE, Murray MT (eds). Textbook of Natural Medicine. Volume 1. St. Louis: Churchill Livingstone Elsevier, 2006.
9. Sexton K, Callahan MA, Bryan EF. Estimating Exposure and Dose to Characterise Health Risks: The Role of Human Tissue Monitoring in Exposure Assessment. Human Tissue Monitoring and Specimen Banking: Opportunities for Exposure Assessment, Risk Assessment and Epidemiological Research. Research Triangle Park, North Carolina: Environmental Health Perspectives, 1993.

10. Clark NM, Baily WC, Rand C. Advances in Prevention and Education in Lung Disease. American Journal of Respiratory Critical Care Medicine. 1998(157): S155-S67.
11. Smith KR. National burden of disease in India from indoor air pollution. Procedures of the National Academy of Sciences. 2000;97(24):13286-93.
12. Bauld L, Chesterman J, Judge K, Pound E, Coleman T. Impact of UK National Health Service smoking cessation services: variations in outcomes in England. Tobacco control. 2003(12):296-301.
13. Lowry S. Sources and effects of indoor air pollution. British Medical Journal. 1989; 299:1388-90.
14. Fergusen EC, Maheswaran R, Daly M. Road-traffic pollution and asthma - using modelled exposure assessment for routine public health surveillance. International Journal of Health Geographics. Volume 3, 2004.
15. Taylor D. Seeing the forests for more than the trees. Environmental Health Perspectives. 1997;105(11):1186-91.
16. Aladag N, Filiz TM, Topsever P, Gorpelioglu S. Parents' knowledge and behaviour concerning sunning their babies; a cross-sectional descriptive study. Biomed Central Pediatrics. Volume 6, 2006.
17. Thiel RJ. Naturopathy For The 21st Century. Warsaw: Wendell W Whitman Company; 2000.
18. Bradley RS. Philosophy of Natural Medicine. In: Pizzorno JE, Murray MT (eds). The Textbook of Natural Medicine. 3rd ed. Volume 1. St Louis: Churchill Livingstone Elsevier, 2006.
19. Ness AR, Frankel SJ, Gunnell DJ, Smith GD. Are we really dying for a tan? British Medical Journal. 1999; 319:113-6.
20. Hollick MF. Resurrection of vitamin D deficiency and rickets. The Journal of Clinical Investigation. 2006;116(8):2062-72.
21. Schauss AG. Suggested Optimum Nutrient Intake of Vitamins Minerals and Trace Elements. In: Pizzorno JE, Murray MT (eds). Textbook of Natural Medicine. 3rd ed. Volume 1. St. Louis: Churchill Livingstone Elsevier, 2006.
22. Dixon ASJ. Health of the Nation and Osteoporosis. Annals of the Rheumatic Diseases. 1992; 51:914-8.

23. Murray MT, Bongiorno PB. Affective Disorders. In: Pizzorno JE, Murray MT (eds). Textbook of Natural Medicine. 3rd ed. Volume 2. St Louis: Churchill Livingstone Elsevier, 2006.

24. Gonzalez H, Tarras-Wahlberg N, Stromdahl B, et al. Photostability of commercial sunscreens upon sun exposure and irradiation by ultraviolet lamps. Biomed Central Dermatology. Volume 7, 2007.

LEARNING SESSION NINE: ENERGY, BODY COMPOSITION AND WEIGHT

Introduction

In this session, we discover what it is that our body does with the food we eat, how energy is generated in the body's cells and what happens to the excess we take in. We look at foods that sap our energy and those that give us a boost and the effect that sugar consumption has on energy levels, short and long-term. We also look at the issue of calories, what they are, what they do and how important or unimportant the actual calorie count of food might be. Do the calories really matter, or does quality triumph over quantity? We also discover the difference between body weight and body composition and what it is we are actually weighing when we step on to the scale.

We then move on to us as an individual, how can we tell what is best for us? How do we make decisions about our own health and food intake as an individual? There are plenty of diets around, but should we be following these and what we are actually losing when we lose 'weight'? We look at body mass index and individual requirements which we will use in the following session to discover how to put on and lose body fat safely and effectively.

We will then come to the fun bit, working it all out in our learning together activities where we will discover just what our requirements really are and how much we can DIY our own programme without fuss and complications. All you need is a pocket calculator, tape measure and pencil. Finally, our discussion session looks at models; midriff and the media! Is there anyone 'normal' still out there? From the size zero to the obesity explosion, have we truly lost the plot or are we being battered into shape?

The Body's Cells: Energy Factories

Plants use the green pigment chlorophyll to trap energy from sunlight. As humans and animals do not have this our only source of energy is food, which requires to be broken down into the essential nutrients. Food passes through the gastrointestinal system where it is broken down by digestive enzymes along the way in a process referred to as digestion. Nutrients are then carried from the small intestine and pass into the bloodstream where they are transported to the individual cells, this whole process is called absorption [1]. The products that reach the cell wall are [1]:

Monosaccharides	Vitamins
Fatty Acids	Minerals
Glycerol	Water
Monoglycerides	Oxygen
Amino Acids	

It helps to think of the cells of the body as individual factories or manufacturing plants. In a very simplified way, this is exactly what they are, raw materials and manufacturing supplies come into the cell like any other factory operation and finished goods and waste materials are secreted out of it. One of three things can happen to the products going into the cell:

a) These essential nutrients may be used as they are to supply energy for the work of other cells in the body, in particular, the heart, lungs, muscles and moving parts;

b) The nutrients may be re-combined to make all the non-essential nutrients that, in turn, make up the building blocks of other chemical components of our cells and tissues, or chemicals such as hormones, which act as messengers telling other cells what to do or enzymes, which speed up reactions;

c) They may be stored for future use in the liver in the form of glycogen, as is the case with glucose, or converted into fats as is the case with unused excessive monosaccharides, or as they are which is the case with fatty acids and stored in special storage units called adipose cells.

The Factory Cell

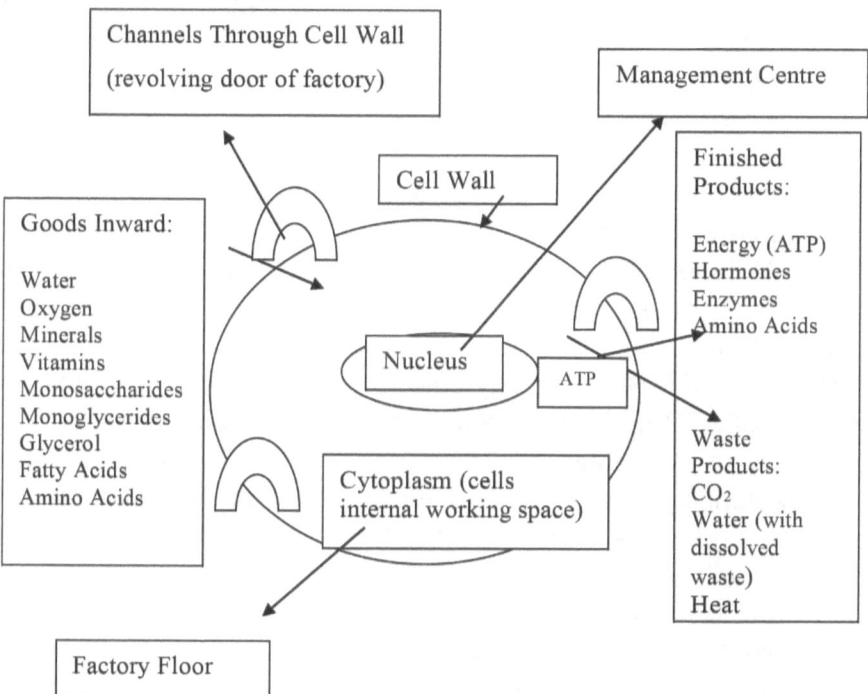

Channels Through Cell Wall (revolving door of factory)

Management Centre

Cell Wall

Finished Products:
Energy (ATP)
Hormones
Enzymes
Amino Acids

Goods Inward:

Water
Oxygen
Minerals
Vitamins
Monosaccharides
Monoglycerides
Glycerol
Fatty Acids
Amino Acids

Nucleus

ATP

Cytoplasm (cells internal working space)

Waste Products:
CO_2
Water (with dissolved waste)
Heat

Factory Floor

Metabolism is the term used for the process by which substances are broken down and re-formed into something else; it is the sum of all the chemical reactions that occur both at the interface of the cell walls and inside the cells of the body. The process of breaking down the raw materials (and used cell parts and waste) is called *catabolism* [1]. The chemical reactions necessary to put together the molecules and simple structures that form the body's tissues and the necessary materials required for their function is called *anabolism* [1]. This is the process whereby the 'finished goods' of the cell are manufactured within it.

The 'finished goods' will be the items necessary for other cells to function as well as the non-essential nutrients. Amino acids and are the principal output as they form the basis of all the enzymes, hormones and the building blocks of new cells. In addition, energy is produced and exchanged. This occurs when the raw materials being broken down undergo *oxidation* which removes electrons from the molecules, thus removing energy from these substances. For this to occur, two B vitamins are necessary, riboflavin and niacin (which temporarily hold on to the energy). This is followed by *reduction* which is the addition of this energy to another molecule which is being formed [1].

The cell itself also needs energy to function. Any left-over energy not required for the next reduction reaction is used to form a molecule called adenosine triphosphate (ATP). In addition, ATP is generated by the oxidation of glucose molecules which releases energy, which in turn is stored in the phosphate bonds of the molecule [1]. ATP is the energy currency of the cell; simply put, the amount of ATP generated represents the amount of energy one has. This is used internally to 'power' the cells break down and manufacturing processes and to 'fuel' the transport of both finished products and waste material across the cell wall into the interstitial fluid. As with any manufacturing process, there is waste which takes the form of carbon dioxide. This is carried in the blood to the lungs to be exhaled and broken-down cell parts which are dissolved in the water of metabolism and carried to the kidneys or liver for processing and excretion in the urine or faeces.

Metabolism is essentially the energy balancing act conducted within the cell that regulates the amount of decomposition (catabolism) with the synthesis (anabolism) of other materials [1]. The metabolic rate is the speed at which these reactions occur; essentially it is how fast and how efficiently our factory cell is running and how much currency (ATP) we have available to spend on running it.

The Fate of Glucose

We now need to think back a little to what happens to the food we consume. Much of the food consumed is in the form of carbohydrates which are broken down in various stages from polysaccharides to simple sugars, monosaccharides, mainly glucose. Fructose and galactose will also be converted into glucose in the liver [1]. Glucose is the preferred source of energy for the body; however, its use depends on the needs of the body cells [1]. Glucose in the cell is used mainly for the generation of ATP, this being the first priority and when there is glucose 'left over' the body has other uses for the excess [1]:

- Some glucose is used in the synthesis of amino acids which are incorporated into proteins.
- Some glucose is stored as glycogen in the liver to act as an emergency energy supply.
- The remainder is converted by the liver into triglycerides and stored as fat in the adipose tissue.

Except for the brain and the liver, all the other body cells rely on *insulin,* a hormone secreted by the pancreas to carry glucose into the cell membranes. When there is more glucose circulating in the blood, the pancreas secretes more insulin, and when there is less glucose in the blood, the pancreas secretes less. Normally this flows smoothly with glucose arriving from the intestines into the bloodstream in a steady slow trickle which the pancreas and circulating insulin can deal with and which the cells can utilise [2]. When a huge load of glucose, however, arrives at once in the form of simple sugars and quickly broken down refined carbohydrates (cola and cake!), the whole process speeds up. Not all parts of the system, however, can cope with this. The pancreas pours out insulin which carries the glucose to the cells, which in turn take what they can use and convert the rest into triglycerides (using up a heck of a lot of spare energy to do it) which are returned to the bloodstream and stored in the adipose tissues. This often leaves circulating insulin in the blood without enough glucose to use it up – hence the body starts asking for more glucose, so one feels hungry, tired, deflated, shaky, light-headed, and in need of something to eat.

In order for all of the cellular functions to occur continuously and to provide the body with all of its requirements, we need all of the essential nutrients to be present in the body at any given time [1]. If some are not available, the cells cannot function effectively or manufacture enough energy. If we add insult to injury by placing a heavy burden of glucose into the system and not enough nutrients, ATP and other products of the cell will not be generated in adequate amounts. We will not dispose of unwanted waste products adequately either [3], and much of the glucose consumed will be converted into adipose tissue [2].

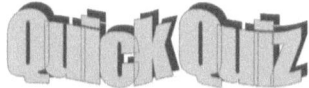

Using coloured pencils to match the foods and drinks on the left to the list of outcomes on the right, what do you think eventually happens to the following:

1.	Chocolate sponge with jam and sweetened whipped cream	A.	Slow burning carbohydrate results in a reasonable, steady trickle of glucose into the cells, giving sustained energy and amino acids which are used for protein synthesis, also some benefit to colon
2.	High fibre sugar free muesli with plain yoghurt	B.	Quick burst of energy from quickly metabolising refined carbohydrate and sugar, some is used but a lot is converted to triglycerides and stored, feeling of hunger after a short time
3.	Bowl of porridge and stewed Apple / applesauce	C.	A mixture of fast burning and refined carbohydrate and sugar with some slowing of digestion due to the presence of fat, the medium flow of glucose into the cell, some moderate excess converted into triglycerides
4.	Doughnut and cola	D.	Slow burning carbohydrate gives sustained trickle of utilisable energy, little left unused

Energy and Calories: Are They Connected?

Energy is defined as "the capacity to do work", the ultimate source of all energy in living organisms is the sun. As we have seen, living plants, intercept this energy, but our own source of energy comes second hand from plants or even 'pre-owned' from herbivorous animals and fish which consume plants. Plants store energy in the chemical bonds of carbohydrates and everything else, proteins and fats are created from this source. Hence it is naturally the human body's preferred source of energy as well. Energy must be supplied regularly to meet the need for the body's survival [4].

As we have seen in the previous section, the food we eat eventually breaks down into glucose and then enters the cells. Energy is released from the molecules of glucose resulting in the creation of ATP and other materials, and the conduction of the body processes such as nerve conduction, enzyme reactions, the mechanical work of muscles and the eventual release of heat to maintain the necessary core temperature of the body. The total amount of energy taken in is important in keeping the body moving, functioning and at the correct temperature for the necessary chemical processes to take place. There is a baseline requirement for energy, below which the metabolic rate (speed of cellular processes) necessary for survival cannot be maintained. This requirement is unique to each individual and is termed the Basal Metabolic Rate (BMR). Several things affect the BMR including gender, age, hormonal status and extremes in ambient temperature [4].

Taking in the right amount of energy is only one-third of the equation in utilising food and maintaining energy levels for work, for this process has two other very important requirements. Just as important as the intake of energy are the intake of nutrients and the rate of energy release from food. In order to be fully utilised the food taken in requires the correct nutrients, in fact, all the essential nutrients, to be present in the body in the minimally required amounts at the same time. This is termed metabolic dependency. If nutrients are missing, food cannot be correctly utilised, and the glucose molecules will not be taken up by the cells, they will be converted into triglycerides instead and stored in the fatty adipose tissue. If the rate of conversion to glucose is too fast and the bloodstream contains too much glucose at once, again only a portion of the glucose will be taken up by the cells and utilised, and the rest will be converted into triglycerides and stored in the adipose tissue [4]. The net result will be a gain in adipose tissue and a loss of potential cellular energy and possibly a slowdown in the conversion of glucose and nutrients into essential finished products of cellular metabolism, such as repair materials, enzymes, proteins and hormones.

Unlike other nutrient requirements, body weight, or more correctly body fat mass, is an indicator of energy adequacy or inadequacy. Since the body has a unique ability to shift the fuel mixture of carbohydrates, proteins and fats to accommodate energy requirements, by converting everything into glucose, there is always a potential for energy requirements to be met. Consuming too little however will always mean insufficiency over a period of time but consuming too much will result in changes in body mass. Although body weight reflects energy intake, what it does not reflect is the adequacy of either macronutrient (protein, fat or carbohydrate) intake or micronutrient intake, and is therefore not an indicator of nutritional status [4].

A calorie is the amount of heat required to raise a single gram of water from 15 °C to 16 °C (i.e. 1 °C). Because the amount of potential energy locked in food is large, the kilocalorie is used to measure it. One kilocalorie (1 kcal) is 1000 calories and is abbreviated to 'C'. The kcal (C) is commonly used to measure the stored energy in food as well as the requirement of the human body for energy. Potentially calories then, are units of energy. So, to go back to the original question: are, energy and calories connected? Well, somewhat, but they are not the same thing, and calories do not automatically translate into immediately utilisable energy. Calories are also not an indicator of how well-nourished one is. As we have seen from the aforementioned information, you can take in a lot of high calorific foods and not gain the energy you require to do the work you would like your body to do, especially when you are nutrient deficient, or taking in the kind of food that translates easily into adipose tissue. As many people have discovered to their discontent, you can put on a significant amount of body fat without gaining a significant amount of instantly utilisable energy, under adverse conditions much of the intake could be stored away [4].

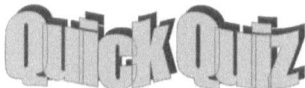

Following is a list of 10 food items which will fall into one of three categories:

a) Slow burning, complex carbohydrate / protein with high micronutrient density, energy sustaining and highly utilisable.

b) Complex carbohydrate which is relatively unrefined and high fibre slowing down the digestion, moderately nutritious and of some use but in excess might be partially converted to triglycerides and stored.

c) Quick burning carbohydrate foods with little fibre or protein, gives a quick energy boost but could lead to a letdown and highly likely to be converted into triglycerides and stored in the adipose tissue.

Match the food to the category you think it falls into:

Food Item   Category

1. Oats porridge with fresh fruit and molasses

2. Lentil and walnut pate with wholegrain toast

3. Organic honey and sesame bar

4. Low fat blueberry muffin with jam

5. Lightly salted bite-sized rice cakes

6. Mixed leaf salad with pimentos and olives

7. Low fat muesli honey biscuits

8. Baked sweet potato with poached egg

9. Ryvita with sugar-free marmalade

10. Homemade vegetable soup with oatcakes

Body Weight and Body Composition

That obesity is on the rise is not new, it was the subject of a WHO report almost a decade ago and has been added to the list of growing concerns internationally. In addition, obesity has now reached epidemic proportions in some countries [5]. Obesity-related disorders include type 2 non-insulin dependent diabetes, hypertension and stroke, coronary artery disease, gallstones [6] and certain cancers [6,7]. Childhood obesity is also a growing concern and children are falling prey to what were previously adult obesity-related problems such as insulin resistance [8]. At the other extreme, some people do not have enough to eat, either unintentionally or due to an eating disorder. In the late 1980's more than 200,000 people were dependent upon charity run soup kitchens in the state of New York USA, [9] a figure which has recently risen to more than 1.5 million. Research into eating disorders estimated that, at any given time, 35% of teenagers in the UK are dieting, whilst in fact, 7-10% are clinically obese, and approximately 1.5% fall into the category of having an eating disorder [10].

To some extent, body image is mediated by culture, with some cultures more concerned about size than others. In multi-ethnic communities, concerns about body mass have been found to be equal in girls of all racial origins; however, the concerns relating to actual dissatisfaction with one's own body shape are not. Despite the same cultural exposure, black and mixed-race girls interviewed in Cape Town have been found to be less dissatisfied with their shape and image than white girls who express far stronger concerns about the way they look. Eating disorders are thought more likely to be culture reactive than culture bound [11].

Despite the concerns of the WHO and those working with eating disorder patients, a survey of 3,416 primary care physicians revealed that, although many stated that they took an interest in the nutritional status of their patients, most did not put the core competencies of nutritional assessment and management into practice. The attitudes and practices surveyed indicated that there is a need for education in nutrition amongst medical students and primary care practitioners [12].

The BMI is a measure of your weight relative to your height; also waist circumference is a measure of abdominal fat. Combining these with information about your additional risk factors yields your risk for developing obesity-associated diseases [13].

Body Mass Index (BMI)

BMI is a reasonably reliable but imperfect indicator of total body fat, which is related to the risk of disease and death. The score is valid for both men and women, but it does have some limits. The limits are [13]:

- It may **overestimate** body fat in athletes and others who have a muscular build.
- It may **underestimate** body fat in older persons and others who have lost muscle mass.

It is therefore not exact as there are other factors concerned with weight that are not taken into consideration. When you weight yourself you weigh all of yourself, that is the bones, muscles, water content of your body and of course the fat, which itself is divided into two kinds of fat: (structural fat which is the layer of fat beneath the epithelium that provides the insulation as well as the cushioning of organs) and the adipose fat, (the actual 'fat banks'). The structural fat is that which one cannot really afford to lose, and it accounts for between 10 and 14% of total body fat for men and 15 and 19 % for women. In order of weight from heaviest to lightest we have:

Muscle and organ weight   Heaviest
Water weight
Bone Weight
Fat weight   Lightest

The amount of fat one has can also be determined by skinfold anthropometry (SFA) which is highly reliable when taken by a person who has been correctly trained to perform the measurements and interpret the results. This involves taking eight skinfold measurements with a special instrument and calculating the average skinfold fat content from which the average body fat percentage is calculated [4]. Initially when we are losing weight, what we are losing is water, and sometimes muscle tissue.

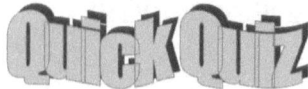

The answers to this quiz really concern only yourself, and you can keep them a secret if you like!

To work out your BMI divide your weight in Kg by your height in Meters squared:

E.g.: Height = 1.68 m and weight 54 Kg
BMI = 54÷ (1.68 x 1.68) = 54 ÷ 2.82 = 19.148 or 19.1

Write Your BMI down here   _____

Determine your waist circumference by placing a measuring tape snugly around your waist. It is a good indicator of your abdominal fat which is another predictor of your risk for developing risk factors for heart disease and other diseases.

Measure in inches or centimetres (1 inch = 2.54 cm)

Write your Waist Measurement down here   _____

A more exact measurement is to divide the hip measurement by the waist measurement.

Write this down here   _____

BMI Score Result

Less than	18.5	Underweight
	18.5 – 24.9	Correct body mass range
	25.0 – 29.9	Overweight
	30.0 +	Obese

Hip to Waist Ratio Result (Risk of Metabolic Syndrome)

Women	Men	
1.4	1.2	Low risk
1.2	1.1	Moderate risk
1.1 or less	1.0 or less	High risk

What is Best for You?

Obesity has been described by the WHO as a global runaway epidemic, no longer confined to the wealthy or older person, which has now reached proportions that require both management and funding strategies [5]. According to the financial institution, Forbes, $46 billion was spent in 2006 alone in the US on diet-related products [14]. For those who are trying to lose weight it may appear that there are a plethora of programmes, but, there are hundreds of diets often based on 'pseudoscience' and dodgy research.

From the point of view of health, it is always best to focus on quality, sustained energy levels and building up resistance to disease by ensuring adequate vitamin intake, especially the antioxidant vitamins [15]! Doing this means, for many people, altering their eating habits over the longer term, in other words, their nutritional lifestyle. As far as altering lifestyle is concerned there are only two types of weight change and health gain programmes around that rely on changes in behaviour. There are those that expect all the changes to be made at once and those that apply a 'stepped care' approach that relies on small changes made at intervals to change long-term lifestyle. It has been found that the former approach only works in the short term and is not easily sustainable and the step by step approach is far more successful over a period of time [16].

Emotions do need to be taken into consideration. Strong emotions are usually connected with the loss of appetite, and reduced food intake, however, in some individuals this does not take place, and their reaction to emotional upset is to eat more. It is generally thought that women are simply more emotional than men, but researchers have found that this is in fact not the case, for women and men are equally upset by adverse events. Women are generally more adept at finding an outlet for emotions even if it is tears and tantrums! People who show their emotions less, however, are more likely to respond to strong emotions by 'comfort eating', or overeating. Amongst people who are obese, the inability to find an emotional outlet is one of the possible causes [17].

Although there are general guidelines, the right weight and the right body proportion for you as an individual will be unique. The amount of energy you need to take in is always linked to your own BMR which can be calculated, in addition to your daily requirements. Your needs for energy will be linked to maintaining, increasing or decreasing your mass and body fat percentage; however one must be careful not to compromise quality to attain a given amount of energy intake.

There are some needs which will be unique to you and some decisions which only you can make for yourself. Ultimately no-one can tell you what is right or wrong; it is a question really of what is right or wrong for you. Ask yourself the following questions:

1. Do I eat when I am angry, unhappy, depressed or bored?
2. Do I eat a lot at once and then try to make up for it by missing the next meal?
3. Do I eat only one meal a day – all day?
4. Do I pick at food that is not particularly nutritious rather than sit down to a meal?
5. Do I eat the right amount of food but not the right kind of food to give myself the nutrients I need?
6. Am I too easily persuaded by others to eat what they want me to eat?
7. Do I sabotage my own nutrition plans when I can see that I am starting to be successful?
8. Do I think I should change the way I eat? (note this is 'should' and not 'can')
9. How much do I really believe that I deserve the best quality of food?
10. Do I think that I deserve to benefit from an improved way of living?

Eating should be a way of life, a joy, a social endeavour and a health-enhancing life-sustaining entity, not a beat yourself up programme!

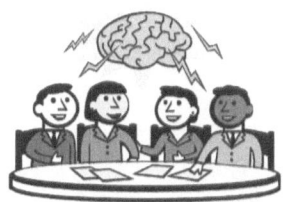

Learning Together

Learning Together

Activity 1: Allow yourselves 10 minutes for this activity

To begin to work out for yourself as an individual your own precise needs, we will look first at the energy requirements and then, over the next few sessions exactly how you can fulfil these to your own benefit. Initially, in small groups working together, we will look at finding each person's unique BMR and the calorific needs that will be required to maintain ones current weight [18].

Technically, men require 1 Cal / Kg per hour, and women require 0.8 Cal / Kg per hour just for baseline survival, that is the energy required to stay alive and breathe slowly (not even opening your eyes as this requires extra energy). In a 24-hour period, this translates into:

For men   BMR = 24 Cal / Kg body mass
For women   BMR = 22 Cal / Kg body mass

To convert imperial weight into metric weight:
Number of whole number stones x 14 + odd no of pounds = total pounds ÷ 2.2 = Kg

Example:
For a woman who is 9 ½ stone 9 x 14 + 7 = 133 pounds ÷ 2.2 = 60.45 Kg
Rounded up or down (in this case down to nearest Kg) = 60 kg x 22 = 1,320 Cal

Now do yours:

Write Your Notes Here

Activity 2: Allow yourselves 15 minutes for this activity

Now taking the BMR requirements, we are going to add to our needs for two types of activity. Firstly, there are those we cannot get away from, i.e. dressing, showering, cooking and a little light housework as well, of course, shopping for food. Then there are those we might choose to do for pleasure, such as playing a sport or going for a walk. For each person in the group follow the steps given:

Cal required for BMR Maintenance _____

Go to the table marked 'Table of Calories Required for Daily Activities':

Now look at the time you take for the following:

Add on:

Activity	Cal/Min	Number of Mins	Total Cal Used
Sleeping			
Showering and personal care			
Food preparation and eating			
Housework			
Driving or walking to work			
Working			
Sub Total			_____

Now add on any other sporting exercising activities you do:

Activity 1
Activity 2
Activity 3

Total needs   _____

Now hang on to this figure as we will need it in the following learning session!

Write Your Notes Here

Now you should take 5 minutes to discuss the results of your learning activities with your facilitator

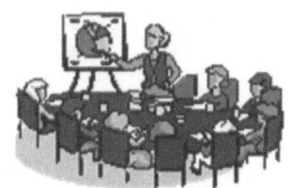

Discussion

Today's Topic for Discussion is: MODELS; MIDRIFF AND THE MEDIA: HAVE WE TRULY LOST THE PLOT OR ARE WE BEING BATTERED INTO SHAPE?

The eating disorders anorexia nervosa and bulimia nervosa comprise a range of physical, psychological and behavioural features. Usually, they have an impact on

social functioning, and their effects pervade most areas of a young person's life. In anorexia nervosa, body weight is maintained at least 15% below that expected.

Weight loss (or failure to increase weight with age) is achieved by restriction of calorific foods, exercise, vomiting or purging. In bulimia nervosa, a persistent preoccupation with eating is present, with craving and consequent binges (often with a subjective feeling of loss of control). Weight is maintained within a normal range by compensatory vomiting or purging. In both conditions, a distortion of body image is present, manifest as a dread of fatness [19,20]. The WHO is equally concerned with the other end of this extreme as deaths due to the complications of obesity resulting in metabolic syndrome, cardiac disorders and stroke, adult onset diabetes mellitus and infective cellulitis continue to rise [5]. The latter problems, however, are no longer confined to chronically overweight adults but have become endemic amongst children in Westernised societies [8]. Meanwhile, we are at the mercy of the media as size zero models strut the catwalk.

Some questions to think about and discuss as a group:

- Should quantity ever be considered before the quality of our food intake?
- How much, if anything, should one be spending on a regular basis on altering one's size or shape?
- Which is more important, health, happiness or looks?
- Does being the best person, we can be, mean conforming to someone else's expectations about our size or shape?

<u>You Might Like to Make Some Notes Here</u>

© A. A. Morris-Paxton 2019

Table of Calories Required for Daily Activities Over and above the BMR Requirement

Activity   **Calories/kg Body Weight/Minute**

	Men	Women
Sleeping	0.1	0.08
Sitting and studying/reading/desk work	0.7	0.6
Cooking food preparation and eating	1.4	1.1
Showering, dressing and personal care	1.5	1.2
Light housework	1.9	1.5
Stretching/Yoga	2.6	2.1
Walk – gentle	2.6	2.1
Light stationery rowing	3.7	3.0
Aerobics (water)	4.2	3.4
Walk - brisk aerobic	4.4	3.5
Aerobics (low impact)	5.3	4.2
Soccer (casual game beach or 5 a side)	7.4	5.9
Swimming moderate freestyle	7.4	5.9
Running (5m/h)	8.4	6.7
Cycling - moderate	8.4	6.7
Circuit training	8.4	6.7
Skipping / jump rope – moderate	10.5	8.4

Adapted and re-worked from information found in: Caloric Expenditure Worksheet for Various Exercise Activities Based on Body Weight HealtheTech Inc., Golden, Co in Krause's Food, Nutrition and Diet Therapy 11th Ed L Kathleen Mahan and Sylvia Escott-Stump, Philadelphia, Saunders Elsevier (2004) and Nutrition Throughout the Life Cycle, Bonnie S Worthington-Roberts and Sue Rodwell Williams McGraw Hill (1999).

References

1. Tortora GJ, Derrickson B. Principles of Anatomy and Physiology. 11 ed. Hoboken: John Wiley & Sons Inc.; 2006.
2. Ettinger S. Macronutrients: Carbohydrates, Proteins and Lipids. In: Mahan LK, Escott-Stump S (eds). Krause's Food Nutrition & Diet Therapy. 11th ed. Philadelphia: Saunders Elsevier, 2004.
3. Plaskett LG. The Wherewithal to Detoxify. Nutrition Information Services 2003.
4. Frary CD, Johnson RK. Energy. In: Mahan LK, Escott-Stump S (eds). Krause's Food Nutrition & Diet Therapy. 11th ed. Philadelphia: Saunders Elsevier, 2004.
5. WHO. Obesity: preventing and managing the global epidemic. Geneva: World Health Organisation, 1998.
6. Sheperd TM. Effective Management of Obesity. The Journal of Family Medicine. 2003;53(1):34-42.
7. Food, Nutrition and the Prevention of Cancer, a Global Perspective. Washington DC: World Cancer Research Fund / American Institute for Cancer Research, 1997.
8. Yensel C, Homme DP, Curry DM. Childhood Obesity and Insulin-Resistant Syndrome. Journal of Pediatric Nursing. 2004;19(4):238-327.
9. Rauschenbach BS, Frongillo EA, Thompson FE, Andersen EJY, Spicer DA. Dependency on Soup Kitchens in Urban Areas of New York State. American Journal of Public Health. 1990; 80:57-60.
10. Nicholls D, Vilner R. Eating Disorders and Weight Problems. British Medical Journal. 2005; 330:950-3.
11. Caradas AA, Lambert EV, Charlton KE. An ethnic comparison of eating attitudes and associated body image concerns in adolescent South African schoolgirls. Journal of Human Nutrition and Dietetics. 2001; 14:111-20.
12. Levin BS, Wigren MM, Chapman DS, Kerner JF, Bergman RL, Rivlin RS. A national survey of attitudes and practices of primary-care physicians relating to nutrition: strategies for enhancing the use of clinical nutrition in medical practice. The American Journal of Clinical Nutrition. 1993; 57:115-9.

13. NIH. Body Mass Index Calculations. US Department of Health and Human Services National Institutes of Health, 2005 Body Mass Index Calculations.
14. Hoffmann L, Rose L. What 10 Diet Plans Cost. New York: Morningstar Inc, 2007.
15. Fletcher RH, Fairfield KM. Vitamins for Chronic Disease Prevention in Adults. Journal of the American Medical Association. 2002;287(23):3127-9.
16. Carels RA, Darby L, Cacciapaglia HM, et al. Applying a stepped-care approach to the treatment of obesity. Journal of Psychosomatic Research. 2005; 59:375-83.
17. Larsen JK, Strien TV, Eisinga R, Engels RCME. Gender differences in the association between alexithymia and emotional eating in obese individuals. Journal of Psychosomatic Research. 2006; 60:237-43.
18. Schultz B. Basal Metabolic Rate (BMR), Energy Expenditure and Body Composition Accessed 2007 May 2007. Cornel University, 2006.
19. Gowers SG. Evidence Based Research in CBT with Adolescent Eating Disorders. Child and Adolescent Mental Health. 2006;11(1):9-12.
20. WHO. The International Classification of Mental and Behavioural Disorders 10th Revision. Geneva: World Health Organisation, 1992.

LEARNING SESSION TEN: PUTTING THE NUTRIENTS TOGETHER

Introduction

This section follows directly on from the end of the last one and looks at our individual needs and how we can fulfil them. In addition, we combine all of the knowledge that we have gained so far in this programme. We learn about creating our own nutritional programme, and we discover in this session the tools we can use to put our new-found knowledge and understanding together.

We explore the use of various designs of the food pyramids, food exchange lists, and the advantages and considerations of these. We also explore, the 'colour wheel', and how the focus of this and the other tools differ according to the aims of their use. We then move on to explore portions, sizes and what constitutes an item of food or a food exchange.

The timing of foods, meals and snacks is looked at as well as how this affects how our body uses food. In addition, we gain an understanding of why breakfast is so important and how to get over the problem of that feeling of 'just can't face it' early morning lack of appetite. Finally, we take a look briefly at exercise and how to use a safe (cheap) easy and effective gradated programme to change the body we've got into to the body we want. The all-important issue of common sense rounds up this session before we move on to the learning together exercises.

Today we are going to choose our own tools and reminder cards! After this we move on to ask the question, do we love ourselves or don't we? The topic of our discussion today is the question of knowing one's own worth. How much are you worth and are you giving yourself all you deserve?

Using Tools in a Nutritional Programme

Individual health behaviours, which include nutrition and exercise, are the products of a complex interweaving of biographical, social and cultural factors. It is therefore important to consider such factors when contemplating any health-related change. Factors that contribute to individual health-related practice, such as what one may or may not eat, fall into three categories [1]:

- Predisposing factors: knowledge, beliefs, values, attitudes
- Enabling factors: availability and accessibility of health resources, education community support and commitment to health, health-related skills
- Reinforcing factors: family, friends, employer, and health provider

Creating your own nutritional programme is not as difficult as it sounds, and it will be of added benefit in that it is one that is right for you and takes into consideration your own circumstances, lifestyle, culture and resources.

Predisposing Factors

Such factors include not only the knowledge gained through your current participation in this programme but also the cultural knowledge that you have brought with you and the eating practices that are common in your own culture. When making decisions about food, one either consciously or unconsciously asks two questions [2]:

- Is it safe to eat?
- Is it good for me?

The question of safety arises because plants may inherently have certain toxins that are poisonous to animals, thus naturally ensuring the plants' survival and evolution. Even when not poisonous, certain parts of plants may be more acceptable in some cultures than in others, and every culture will have its own way of preparing these items for eating [2]. The question of 'goodness' or benefit to health also arises as knowledge passed down the generations of what makes a person feel good or ill, or helps heal certain ailments, will also form part of the cultural cuisine. Sometimes such knowledge is helpful and has been recently scientifically verified. Sometimes this is not helpful and is borne of myth rather than fact [2].

Enabling Factors

There has been a significant disparity in health education, access to health education and resources to enable people to access health care programmes which the US government is attempting to deal with in their goals for 'healthy people 2010'. This programme goes part way into redressing some of these issues; however, people themselves need to exercise their right to equal health care and support one another as a community [3]. An Australian study found that community support and community-based programmes have been of great value in enhancing health. It has been proposed that community-based action, peer support and social marketing of the benefits of good nutrition may be the way of the future in disease prevention [4,5].

Reinforcing Factors: Tools We Use

More than 40 nutrients are required in the human diet, and the only sure way of getting all of them in a reasonably utilisable quantity is to have as wide a variety of foods that have been as minimally processed and refined as possible [2]. Advertising has a huge impact on what we buy, and there have never been so many food choices available [5], the problem being that many of these items are made up of similar ingredients thus even with a large choice available the ingredients may limit the dietary intake. Social marketing, however, can be a force for good when healthy eating habits are reinforced. Research has found that with awareness and enhanced knowledge, even eating out can be healthy [5].

Numerous standards serve as a guide for both evaluating current national food intakes and planning and evaluating diets of both individuals and groups of people. Many countries have issued national guidelines which they believe appropriate for the circumstances and needs of their respective populations [6]. There are some helpful tools that aid in planning a nutritional programme and reminding us of what our intake should ideally be which have for many years, been available to dieticians. More recently some have now been revamped and made available in two forms to the public, Among these are various versions of the food pyramid and food exchange systems that we will now discuss [6].

The Food Pyramid

Various countries, including the UK, US, Canada and Australia, have food guide pyramids. Essentially these translate the national dietary guidelines and nutritional recommendations of the country into a visual form that is user-friendly.

The US Food Pyramid:

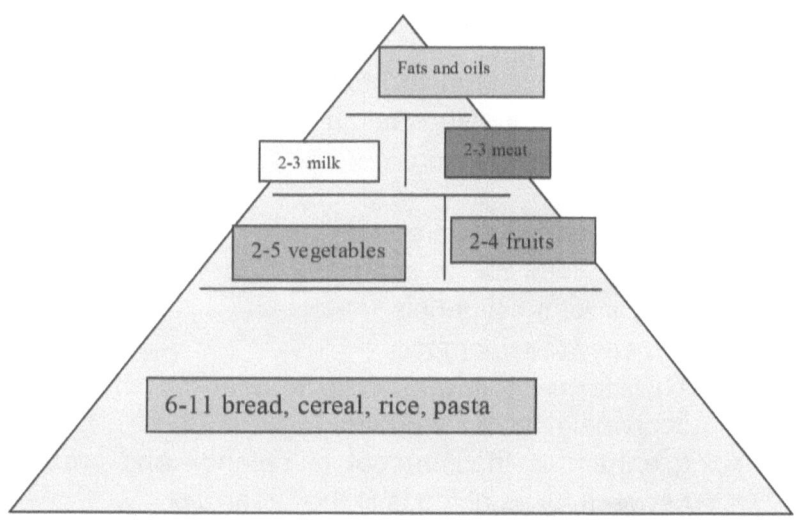

Adapted from: The Food Guide Pyramid US Department of Agriculture and US Department of Health and Human Services [7].

The Children's version of this same pyramid allows for 6 servings of bread and cereals, 3 vegetables, 2 fruits, 2 portions of milk, 2 portions of meat and sparing amounts of fats and sweets [6].

Canada's food guide to healthy eating constitutes a rainbow with four food groups:

The Food Guide Rainbow

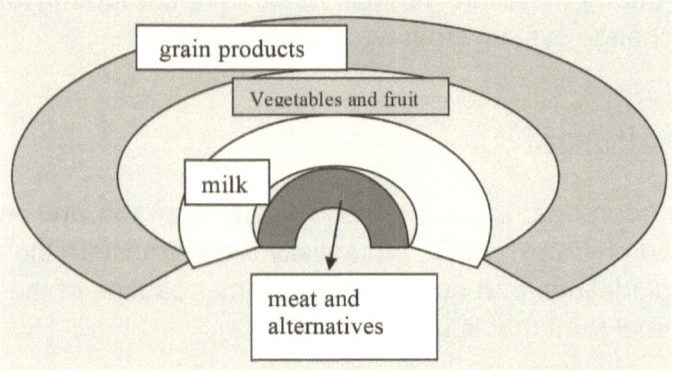

Adapted from: Canada's Food Guide to Healthy Eating, the Office of Nutrition Policy and Promotion, Health Canada, 2002[8]

Both schemes are built from the food exchange system which we will discuss in the next subsection, and both have significant advantages as well as some considerations:

- The main advantages are:
  - Viewing information in a pictorial form tends to make it clearer for most people
  - It is easy to remember
  - This form of information is user-friendly and not overwhelming or off-putting
  - It enhances the concept of balance and proportion between types of foods in the 'ideal' diet
- The main considerations are:
  - There is no international consistency, and there are different versions of the food pyramid in different countries

- Commercial sponsorship is often involved in the advertising of the food pyramids that influence what type of foods are given as examples
- There is no distinction between whole foods and processed foods (between white and whole grain bread for example).
- In some pyramids (the UK) and the Canadian rainbow concept, there are no guidelines given as to the proportion of fruit to vegetables recommended, and they are viewed as a single food group despite having differing carbohydrate components and different types of micronutrient content.

The Food Exchanges

Many food guides and other recommendations emphasise eating a wide variety of foods to achieve dietary adequacy. According to the US Food and Nutrition Board, choosing various foods to meet the dietary recommendations should, in theory, provide adequate amounts of the nutrients that do not have well defined recommended levels. A varied diet also ensures that sufficient amounts of substances, such as fibre and phytonutrients that are not defined officially as nutrients but may influence health, are also taken in. It appears that increasing the number of different foods eaten over a period of time improves food choices in general [6].

The above guides were developed from the food exchange system which is used internationally. The food exchange system standardises serving sizes and is set by governments based on reference amounts commonly consumed. Food exchange systems commonly categorise foods by macronutrient category and calorie / energy content [9]:

Starch Exchanges 15 g carbohydrate, 3 g protein, 0-1 g, fat 80 calories
        Includes grains and cereals, starchy vegetables,
        beans, peas and winter squashes such as pumpkins

Other carbohydrate foods 15 g carbohydrate, 3-8 g protein, 0-8 g fat
Includes cakes, biscuits and cereal bars, ice cream
and desserts

Fruit Exchanges 15 g carbohydrate 60 calories
Includes all fruit and fruit juices

Milk Exchanges 12 g carbohydrate, 8 g protein, 0-8 g fat, 90-150 calories
Includes all milk-based foods and soy milk

Meat Exchanges 0 g carbohydrate, 7 g protein, 3-5 g fat, 55-75 calories
Includes chicken, fish, all meat products eggs and
cheeses

Fat Exchanges 5 g fat, 45 calories
Includes oils, spreads, avocado, nuts, seeds and
salad dressings

Many diet club plans such as Weight Watchers International, Weigh Less, and others work on a version of the food exchange system converted into points, sins, counts or similar measuring techniques for the exchanges one consumes. Mainly, such programmes focus on macronutrients and calories. To their credit, however, an abundance of fruits and vegetables are encouraged, and fats are limited.

The Colour Wheel

This is developed from the recommendations of the Food and Agricultural Organisation (FAO) and the WHO and gives a guide on what you can eat and should be eating and not on what you should not be eating. It focuses on the ratio of macronutrients as well as obtaining the minimum micronutrients. The secret of the colour wheel is that it looks at proportions; therefore your diet cannot get out of balance. It works by not only looking at the correct ratios of carbohydrate to protein to fat but also at the requirements for fat-soluble and water-soluble nutrients, omega ω3: ω6: ω9 and the storage and self-manufacturing capabilities of the body for nutrients.

The Colour Wheel

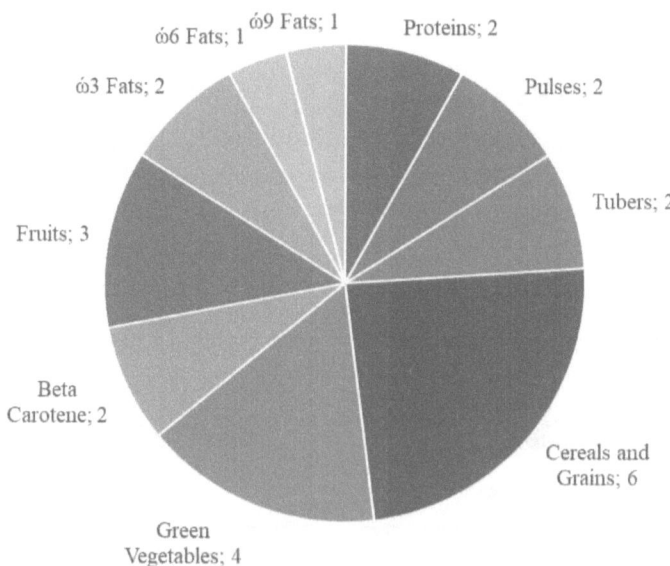

NB: This chart gives the ratio of ώ6: ώ3: ώ9 as 1:2:1 and in session 2 it was recommended that one takes in the ratio 3:1:1. One should be aware that there is also considerable ώ6 fatty acid content in the proteins of animal origin such as meats, chicken and dairy products as well as ώ3 in fish.

The colour wheel is much more structured than other food guides and attempts to focus on nutrition as opposed to weight, or calories. This chart is not commercially influenced and is based on the Food and Agricultural Organisation and WHO guidelines for the minimum requirements for adults for energy, protein and nutrients. The focus is on providing enough micronutrients for the prevention of chronic diseases and the maintenance of health as opposed to losing weight or controlling calories [10]. It aims to meet the recommendations of the WHO by increasing the intake of fruits and vegetables, increasing the intake of fish and ώ3 fatty acids and changing the types of fats and the ratios of fats consumed. This particular guide also aims to decrease and discourage the use of other animal proteins, especially red meats, as per WHO recommendations [10].

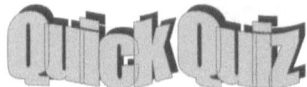

You have been given some possible advantages and considerations of using various food guides for daily living. Working in small groups and avoiding the ones already given, can you add to this information by looking at your own lives and deciding on:

1. An extra possible advantage of using the food pyramid:

    _____

    _____

2. An extra possible consideration of using the food pyramid:

    _____

    _____

3. An extra possible advantage of using the food rainbow:

    _____

    _____

4. An extra possible consideration of using the food rainbow

    _____

    _____

5. On a scale of 1 (not at all user friendly) to 10 very user friendly how do you rate the food exchange system?

    _____

    _____

6. Why?

    _____

    _____

7. There have been no advantages or considerations given for 'The Colour Wheel' Can you think of a) an advantage? b) a consideration?

Portions and Sizes: How Much is 'One'?

Standard serving sizes of foods are set by governments, based usually on reference amounts of foods commonly consumed by the general public [6]. This means that what is consumed in a given population is taken as a reference amount for comparison of nutritional values as opposed to what ought to be consumed. In addition, in different countries, there will be varying ideas of what a commonly consumed amount is and different cultures within a given country may or may not consider that same amount of food 'a portion'.

Nutrition fact labels are slightly more helpful in that they give the nutritional values per portion as well as defining what the manufacturer means by 'a portion,' i.e. ½ can or 100 g or 2 crackers etc. Often the percentage of a nutrient in relation to the daily value or recommended amount is given in addition. As this one nutritional standard may not apply to everyone, however, this may not be a useful measure [6].

How much a portion is depends on who is measuring the portion and what is being measured. Since the government tends to take 'typically eaten' portions as a standard measure, this may well change with circumstances. Research has shown that when we are exposed to education and made aware of the importance of fruit and vegetables, as well as having a little motivation, people ate more fruit and vegetables. Not only was an increased variety consumed but also the quantity was increased [11]. A portion, therefore, can be quite literally 'a moveable feast'. Calls have been made for changes in food labelling and for increased awareness of the quality of foods consumed as opposed to the quantity. In order to meet the 2010 goals for Healthy People, some scientists feel that there should be a greater emphasis on the consumption of fresh foods and unrefined foods, rather than the reliance on portion sizes [12].

The group of international scientists who produced the expert report for the WHO/ FAO have also recommended a change in emphasis globally, from recommendations which are restrictive and calorie / food exchange based, to ones which are based on the quality of intake and are likely to fulfil micronutrient requirements [10]. This means, in effect, that it might be better to define a portion as the practically consumable amount of a given food that would contain a useful quantity of micronutrients.

The food pyramids, food rainbow and the food exchange list, focus on a specific calorific value as well as the macronutrient content for a portion of food but are not always realistic, i.e. ¼ bagel equals one starch exchange or one cereal portion. This might not be very useful when deciding whether to eat a bagel. Does one eat the bagel (4 exchanges of starch) or go without, or eat something else? If the bagel is made from white bread flour one might be in danger of using ones 'starch allowance' without obtaining enough B-complex vitamins, fibre, magnesium or other minerals.

The number of portions in the colour wheel is based on a reasonable edible portion of unprocessed micronutrient dense food and taken together will provide between 1,600 and 2,100 Calories per day. Below the 1,600 Calorie mark, it is extremely difficult, if not impossible to construct a diet which can provide the essential nutrients for a healthy adult without compromising health, or necessitating the intake of supplements [13].

Recommended as one portion:

Food	Size	Amount
Fruit (fresh)	Large fruits: apples, pears, peaches, nectarines	1 medium
	Small fruits: plums apricots dates and figs	2 medium
	Small melon or large banana	1/2
	Berries and cut fruit	½ cup
Beta-carotene	Large carrots	1
	Pumpkin, winter squash	½ cup
	Cantaloupe, papaya	½ medium

Leafy green vegetables	Small size or chopped vegetables	½ cup <u>minimum (there are no maximum quantities)</u>
	Florets, cabbage or lettuce	1 cup or ¼ head <u>minimum</u>
Cereal and grains	Whole grain bread, pumpernickel, small whole wheat pita, roll or pancake	1 slice or 1 single
	Rice, millet, couscous, bulgur, buckwheat, oats	½ cup cooked (1/4 cup uncooked)
	Whole grain unsweetened breakfast cereals	½ cup
Tubers	Large: mature potatoes, yams	1 small / ½ cup / 3 slices
	New potatoes, turnips, parsnips, beets	2 medium
Pulses	Fresh: peas, broad beans or dried, cooked beans, lentils or chickpeas Soya milk or yoghurt	½ cup cooked (¼ cup dry uncooked) ½ cup
Proteins	Sardines / pilchards	2 canned /1 large fresh
	Salmon, tuna, mackerel other white fish	¼ can drained ½ small fillet
	Chicken, turkey or game	2 small slices roast
	Egg – medium Milk Cottage cheese	1 whole 1/3 cup ¼ cup
	Mycoprotein / TVP	1 small piece / 2 slices / ¼ cup dried
ὠ 3 Fats	Walnut (English) halves Linseeds, pumpkin seeds	4 large 1 Tbs.
ὠ 6 Fats	Almonds, cashews, Peanut butter or tahini Avocado pear	6 2 tsp ¼ fresh
ὠ 9 Fats	Olives Olive or canola oil	8 1 tsp

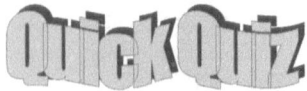

Look at the list below and based on the information you now have:

1. Circle in green the portions of food you feel are appropriate

2. Circle in red the portions of food you feel are too large to be a single portion

3. Circle in yellow the portions of food you feel are too small to be realistic

4. Circle in blue the portions of food you feel do not contain enough micronutrients to warrant being included in nutrition guidelines

A medium turkey drumstick   ½ pita bread   1 medium slice rye bread

1 small box of salted, buttered popcorn   ¼ large waffle

1 T-bone steak   1 small packet wine-gums   ½ large baked potato

½ cup rice and millet flakes   ½ small roast chicken

¼ bagel   2 squares of chocolate   1 small candyfloss

2 beef sausages   ½ cup chopped lettuce

1 large grated carrot   8 black olives   2 tsp cream

1 fried cod fillet   1 cup instant pudding

Timing Meals and the Importance of Breakfast

The body's metabolism is like a well-run machine when it has fuel that is. Like any other piece of complex equipment, it cannot run effectively on empty and given nothing, for long enough it, of course, will not run at all. The metabolism is connected to one's own biorhythms which in turn are connected to the pattern of light and dark. During darkness, the body naturally slows down the processes of building energy and begins to repair, grow new cells and detoxify the system. As the light slowly begins to affect the system, these processes come to an end, and the business of creating energy for work begins [14].

Originally the eating pattern of humans was to gather food throughout the day, hunting (mainly fish) in the months when nuts, berries and roots were more scarce [15,16]. The metabolism was built for a mainly plant-based diet, high in dietary fibre with occasional animal products, eaten in small manageable amounts on a frequent basis [15]. There is no evidence to the contrary; things have not suddenly changed just because of commuting, office hours, or cafeteria opening times.

The ideal time to consume food it would appear is during the daylight hours and on a regular ongoing basis. The more frequently one eats, the better the body can burn the food, control the steady flow of glucose into the bloodstream and utilise the nutrients and provide us with sustained energy. In addition, taking in whole, unprocessed foods of vegetable origin with a good measure of fibre / NSP has been shown to prevent excessive circulating glucose concentrations and thus also prevent high amounts of circulating insulin which carry this glucose into the adipose tissue. This, in turn, has been shown not only to decrease fat deposition but data indicate that replacement of 5.4% of total dietary carbohydrate with NSP significantly increased lipid oxidation and therefore could decrease fat accumulation in the long-term [17].

Breakfast is critical to metabolism, and without breakfast the metabolic rate drops, leading to impaired usage of a normal calorific amount of food. In effect, the less one eats particularly early in the day, the more the body compensates by lowering the requirement for calories by slowing down the metabolic rate. Unfortunately, this also slows down the rate of repair of tissues and the rate of build-up of immune resources.

In addition, depression, decreased resistance to stress and cold as well as an increased propensity to illness and higher BMI with an increased propensity to obesity has been found in those who either skipped breakfast completely or ate breakfast on an irregular basis [18]. The effect of starting school or work without breakfast is costly and has been shown to affect the results of school tests quite adversely [19]. Research has demonstrated that not eating breakfast results in a lowered ability to take in and process information. More mistakes are made in completing complex tasks, decision making and recall of information [19].

Some people, however, feel that they cannot eat breakfast and are simply not hungry in the morning. This could be due to several factors that have nothing to do with breakfast per se but could be because one has eaten late the previous night and has not digested their food. If one has a pattern of going hungry all day and only eating one large meal at night, there is not enough energy to digest that meal and not enough digestive enzymes either. This leads to food leaving the stomach and gastrointestinal system more slowly. Thus it might only be the next morning before this process is complete, hence one is not hungry. This could turn into a vicious cycle, resulting in low energy levels and obesity. To break the pattern, it would be best to choose one day when one does not eat at night, takes in plenty of fluids and begins again fresh the next morning with a light breakfast.

Other solutions include:

- Beginning with fresh fruit which metabolises quickly and following this with a high fibre cereal 2-3 hours later
- Beginning with a blender breakfast of fresh fruit and yoghurt which contains a mixture of medium glycaemic and low

glycaemic foods as well as bifidoflora which help complete digestion in the lower intestine

- Beginning with water and fresh juice and then going for a pre-breakfast walk to encourage an increase in metabolism and build up an appetite

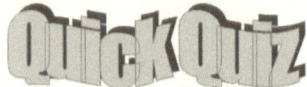

Look at the list below and, based on the information you now have:

a) Underline in green the breakfasts you feel might be appropriate for someone with little early morning appetite or not used to eating breakfast

b) Underline in red the meals that you feel are too large or unsuitable for breakfast

c) Underline in yellow the breakfast items that are realistic for someone on a healthy nutrition programme that has a reasonable appetite

d) Underline in blue the breakfasts that are light, if one has little appetite but not very nutritious

1. Two fried eggs, bacon, sausage and chips

2. Muesli with plain yoghurt and a piece of chopped fresh fruit

3. Fresh orange juice and a small bowl of stewed apple

4. Two chocolate digestive biscuits and a cup of tea/coffee with milk and sugar

5. Blended banana with apple juice and yoghurt

6. Three egg, cheese and onion omelette, fried tomato and French toast

7. A caramel cereal bar and orangeade

8. Two slices of wholegrain toast with unsweetened peanut butter and applesauce

Finding the Right Balance for You

In addition to the dietary tools that we have looked at and the timing of meals, there are other components to finding the right balance of food and lifestyle, such as exercise, convenience and common sense. The 2006 version of the US food pyramid includes exercise as part of the daily programme; however, it gives no guidelines as to how much or what type. Without structured guidelines, this might be a two-edged sword, as too much exercise too soon can also be damaging. Clearly, there are physical, psychological and stress relieving benefits of exercise which can play a role in long-term health maintenance and disease prevention. Long-term maintenance of an exercise programme, however, is every bit as difficult as long-term maintenance of a nutritional programme [20]. The best way to do this is to [21]:

- Find something you like and feel that you can keep up
- Start slowly
- Build up gradually
- Participate with a friend or in a group

Walking has been advocated as the safest, easiest and least expensive, as it combines the benefits of cardiovascular exercise and weight-bearing exercise which tones muscles and increases bone density [21]. Take the following tips:

- Begin with 20 minutes, walk slowly for five, briskly for ten and then slow down for the last five minutes.
- Increase the brisk walk by five minutes every fifth day until you reach 30 minutes of brisk walking (you should be able to maintain this and still talk).
- Next, increase the slow walking for an extra 5 minutes at the beginning and end
- Add on 5 minutes stretching before and after the exercise

Change is not easy we acknowledge this, although it can be made less difficult. There are various stages in changing [22]:

- Pre-contemplation
  - This is the stage of information gathering and feedback, one may or may not feel at this stage that one requires changes to be made
- Contemplation
  - Here one is anticipating improvement and may be aware that some changes could be made
- Preparation
  - This is the planning stage; it is about what changes to make to one's lifestyle and how one might make them
- Action
  - This is the stage at which one actually changes something, builds goals and makes plans for future staged changes
- Maintenance and Lifestyle
  - Changes have been made and have become a part of one's new life.

The chances are that by participating in this programme and having come so far you will be at various stages of the above process with various small changes that you have made, are making or are planning to make.

The Dietary Guidelines Alliance message "It's All About You" reaches out to health consumers motivations, individual needs and life goals and makes the following recommendations [6]:

- Be realistic
  - Make small changes over a period of time in what you eat and what you can do
- Be adventurous
  - Expand your tastes to enjoy a variety of foods
- Be flexible
  - Balance what you eat and what you do over a period of days, do not worry over one meal or one day
- Be sensible

- Bingeing and starving do not serve any purpose if you have a bad day simply acknowledge the fact that it was not your best day, forgive yourself and move on
- Be active
  - Walk the dog or participate in sport, don't just watch it

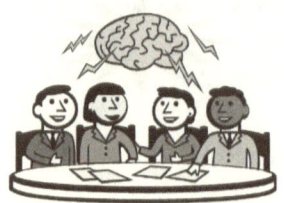

Learning Together

Learning Together

Activity 1: Allow yourselves 15 minutes for this activity

You should know the full total of your needs for calories from the last session. Just to remind yourself write it down here:

My total calorie Requirements are _____

Now look at your needs and ask yourself whether these are more than the minimum 1600 Calories per day or less.

Write the amount by which they are over or
under 1,600 Cal per day _____

If Your Needs are Less do This Section

If your needs are less, the 1 600 calorie minimum then you will still need to eat the minimum amounts in order to nourish yourself, but you could perhaps take more exercise.

Work out the number of calories you need
to walk briskly for one minute for your weight
and multiply this by 5. _____

Now work out how many lots of 5 minutes you
would need to reach the target difference in
calories _____

By increasing your walking for 5 minutes every week, you can get to your goal number of calories to burn without compromising your nutritional status or increasing your body fat.

If Your Needs are More, do This Section

For the first 50 calories over 1,600 choose	1 vegetable
For the next 50 calories over 1,600 choose	1 fruit
For each 100 calories, more than you need add on	1 cereal / grain up to 12 portions
For the following 100 – 200 calories choose either:	1-2 pulses
	1-2 proteins
	1-2 dairy
For the following 100 calories add on	1 ώ6 rich fat plus 1 ώ3 rich fat

Now choose either the basic pyramid; the basic rainbow or the colour wheel and move to the next session

Write Your Notes Here

Activity 2: Allow yourselves 10 minutes for this activity

Now go to the Reminder Sheet (facilitator's handout) for the tool that you have chosen (this will be the rainbow, the pyramid or the colour wheel). The basic requirements for each day have been filled in for you.

1. Add on in the second column any extra daily needs that you have
2. Fill in the total in the next column
3. Multiply by seven to get the weekly total (this is much more practical)
4. Now fill in the weekly total both on your reminder sheet and if you wish on to your pyramid, rainbow or colour wheel.

Write Your Notes Here

Congratulations on having created your own plan your own way! You may take 5 minutes to discuss your results with your facilitator if you wish

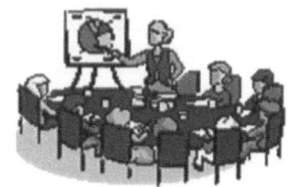

Discussion

Today's Topic for Discussion is: DO YOU KNOW YOUR OWN WORTH AND ARE YOU GIVING YOURSELF ALL YOU DESERVE?

This discussion is about value; how much do we really value ourselves and do we reward ourselves with help or harm? Many people have never been taught to value themselves, worse still they reward themselves with damaging things, which in the extreme version could lead to excessive alcohol intake or recreational drug usage. Often it is damaging foods, those that do nothing for us and might have some taste appeal but detract from our long-term health and happiness.

Some questions to think about and discuss as a group:

- When we reward ourselves for hard work or achievement, how often do we do this with food or drink items as opposed to non-food or drink items?
- If you 'treat' yourself with a large hot chocolate and a piece of rich cake, knowing that there is no long-term benefit, is it really a treat?
- Could this situation fall into a mild 'self-harm' or form of self-sabotage?
- Can we think of items that might be food and drink but are more rewarding nutritionally than damaging?
- Could we feel just as good with a non-food reward such as toiletries, a CD, paperback or movie ticket?
- Could we find a way of celebrating that is not food or drink focussed?

<u>You Might Like to Make Some Notes Here</u>

References

1. Johnson PH, Kittleson MJ. A Qualitative Exploration of Health Behaviours and the Associated Factor among University Students from Different Cultures. The International Electronic Journal of Health Education. Volume 6, 2003:14-25.
2. Truswell AS. ABC of Nutrition: Some Principles. British Medical Journal. 1985; 291:1486-90.
3. Black SA. Diabetes, Diversity and Disparity. American Journal of Public Health. 2002;92(4):543-8.
4. Dunt D, Day N, Pirkis J. Evaluation of a community-based health promotion programme supporting public health policy initiatives for a healthy diet. Health Promotion International. 1999;14(4):317-27.
5. Ancharya RN, Patterson PM, Hill EP, Schmitz TG, Bohm E. An Evaluation of the "TrEAT Yourself Well" Restaurant Nutrition Campaign. Health Education and Behaviour. 2006(June):309-24.
6. Earl R. Guidelines for Dietary Planning. In: Mahan LK, Escott-Stump S (eds). Krause's Food Nutrition & Diet Therapy. 11th ed. Philadelphia: Sunders, 2004.
7. Earl R. The Food Guide Pyramid. US Department of Agriculture and US Department of Health and Human Services, 2004: The Food Guide Pyramid.
8. Earl R. Canada's Food Guide to Healthy Eating. The Office of Nutrition Policy and Promotion: Health Canada, 2004.
9. ADA. Exchange Lists for Meal Planning. American Diabetes Association Inc; American Dietetic Association, 2003.
10. WHO. Diet, Nutrition and the Prevention of Chronic Diseases: Report of a Joint WHO/FAO Expert Consultation. Geneva: World Health Organisation, 2003.
11. Steptoe A, Perkins-Porras L, McKay C, Rink E, Hilton S, Cappuccio FP. Behavioural counselling to increase consumption of fruit and vegetables in low-income adults: randomised trial. British Medical Journal. 2003; 326:855-8.

12. Nestle M, Jacobson MF. Halting the Obesity Epidemic: A Public Health Policy Approach. Public Health Reports. 2000;2000(115):12-24.

13. WHO. Energy and protein requirements report of a joint FAO/WHO/UN expert consultation. Geneva: World Health Organisation, 1985.

14. Beyer PL. Digestion, Absorption, Transport and Excretion of Nutrients. In: Mahan LK, Escott-Stump S (eds). Krause's Food, Nutrition & Diet Therapy. 11th ed. Philadelphia: Saunders Elsevier, 2004.

15. Frassetto L, Morris RC, Sellmeyer DE, Todd K, Sebastian A. Diet, evolution and ageing: The pathophysiological effects of the post-agricultural inversion of potassium-to-sodium and base-to-chloride ratios in the human diet. European Journal of Nutrition. 2001;40(5):200-13.

16. Oppenheimer S. Out of Eden: The peopling of the world. London: Constable and Robinson; 2004.

17. Higgins JA, Higbee DR, Donahoo WT, Brown IL, Bell ML, Bessensen DH. Resistant starch consumption promotes lipid oxidation. Nutrition and Metabolism. Volume 1, 2004.

18. Yang R-J, Wang EK, Hsieh Y-S, Chen M-Y. Irregular breakfast eating and health status among adolescents in Taiwan. Biomed Central Public Health. Volume 6, 2006.

19. Pollitt E, Mathews R. Breakfast and cognition: an integrative summary. American Journal of Clinical Nutrition. 1998;67(S):804.

20. Woodward CM, Berry MJ. Enhancing Adherence to Prescribed Exercise: Structured Behavioural Interventions in Clinical Exercise Programs. Journal of Cardiopulmonary Rehabilitation. 2001; 21:201-9.

21. Lutack B, Bongiorno PB. The Exercise Prescription. In: Pizzorno JE, Murray MT (eds). Textbook of Natural Medicine. 3rd ed. Volume 1. St Louis: Churchill Livingstone Elsevier, 2006.

22. Snetselaar LG. Counselling for Change. In: Mahan LK, Escott-Stump S (eds). Krause's Food Nutrition and Diet Therapy. 11th ed. Philadelphia: Saunders Elsevier, 2004.

LEARNING SESSION ELEVEN: BUILDING RECIPES

Introduction

Everyone has recipes, either from a book or handed down through their family. Alternatively, you may have recipes that you have evolved yourself from ideas you have read about, foods you have eaten in restaurants, or in other people's homes. Some people have their recipes written down whilst others have 'basic ideas' to which are added liberal amounts of herbs, spices, odd items from the fridge and a dash of imagination. Here we look at what we can do with your old recipes, changing ingredients, changing cooking methods and improving on what you already have.

We also look at how you can build new nutritious recipes from the basis of the knowledge you have now acquired and using the tools from the previous session. We discover how we can create our own dietary plan, one that we can enjoy as opposed to one that has been designed by someone else to their own tastes. Most importantly, however, we do not aim to take away your own cultural heritage, this is an important part of who you are. It reflects where you are from, what you believe in, and plays a role in social cohesion, celebration and family life.

We will look at making new recipes from old and explore alternative ways of cooking traditional foods. This session aims to help you build your own programme of health without compromising faith, culture or budget! We look at recipes in three ways, firstly taking what you already have and changing a few ingredients. We then look at increasing the value of what we eat by changing how we prepare it and thirdly we look at building recipes from scratch by looking at our food plan (pyramid, rainbow or 'to whit') and inventing dishes according to our requirements.

Finally, in our learning together sessions, we look at the power of collective input and invent recipes in groups. Following these sessions, our discussion today focuses on the growth of fast food restaurants and the question of eating out vs eating at home and asks: are we witnessing the death of the family dinner?

Converting Recipes and Changing Ingredients

There is not a single diet that is the 'right diet' for everyone. Genetic make-up food allergies and intolerances as well as individual biochemistry, all have an influence on health and food intake [1]. What works for one person does not necessarily work for the next person; hence the guidelines given in the previous session are just that, they are guides, they are not prescriptions. The individual food choices that one makes depend on physiological factors, as well as social, cultural and religious preferences. Society is becoming increasingly multicultural, multi-ethnic and encompasses many different religious beliefs and practices, all of which need to be taken into consideration when planning food, meals and menus [2].

Cultural aspects of food planning and preparation may also include vegetarianism, family heritage and local customs [2]. It is for this reason that actual choices in grains, fruits, vegetables, pulses and other sources of protein can and should remain individual. These are, in part, ones 'comfort zone'. In planning food, one nevertheless has to bear in mind the goals or aims that one is trying to attain, principally those of maintaining health and preventing illness. Several researchers make the following evidence-based recommendations for the prevention of disease [3-6]:

1. Attain and maintain optimal:
    *   Blood glucose levels in the normal range or as close to normal as is possible
    *   Lipid and lipoprotein profile that reduces the risk of vascular disease.
    *   Blood pressure levels that reduce the risk of vascular disease.
2. Modify nutrient intake and lifestyle as appropriate for the prevention and treatment of obesity, inappropriate blood lipid profile, cardiovascular disease and hypertension.

3. Improve health through healthy food choices and physical activity.

4. Address individual nutritional needs, taking into consideration personal and cultural preferences and lifestyle, while respecting the individual's wishes and willingness to change.

These first two aims can be fulfilled with the knowledge you have gained from the previous learning sessions in this programme. We are in the process of fulfilling the third aim between the previous session and this one, as we change what we eat and how we prepare it. The fourth aim really depends on the individual as you can choose to re-create some of your own traditional dishes or ring the changes and try someone else's!

In general, we look first of all at taking any recipe and making the following changes as an initial step to preventing, or mitigating hypertension [3] and carcinogenesis, [5] as well as preventing diabetes and insulin resistance [4,6].

1. Cut down or eliminate the salt and instead increase, or add herbs, lemon or lime juice:
   a. Sweet basil and oregano are good for tomato based and vegetarian dishes.
   b. Rosemary is good for chicken, mushroom or mycoprotein based dishes, as is the combination of sage and chopped onion or shallots.
   c. Thyme is good for meat or TVP based dishes.
   d. Bay is good for dairy, or soymilk-based dishes; sauces, soups and casseroles.
   e. Dill goes well with fish dishes, especially salmon and omega three rich fish.
   f. Parsley goes well with white fish and as an addition to salads and vegetables.
   g. A dash of lemon or lime juice in a soup or casserole just before serving adds vitamin C and potassium and gives it the same tang as would be achieved by adding salt (not recommended for milk-based dishes).

2. Change smoked or cured ingredients for fresh ones and avoid charring:
   a. Lightly grill food indoors and eat 'al fresco' rather than barbecuing outdoors and eating whilst inhaling the wood smoke. If out on a camping site use a portable gas bottle, covered barbecue and cook food in foil (this can be washed, re-used and taken home to dispose of later).

Avoidance of insulin resistance and, blood glucose control in addition to a decrease in risk of cardiovascular disorders [7] can be achieved, in part, by increasing the fibre and micronutrient contents of the diet, making use of the carbohydrate-rich foods, in particular, by making the following changes [6]:

1. Change the refined grains for unprocessed whole grain products:
   a. Change white, wheat-based bread for a wider variety of whole grain bread such as rye bread, pumpernickel, whole wheat pita bread, whole wheat flour tortillas, corn tortillas, multigrain crackers, oatcakes.
   b. Change refined sweetened breakfast cereals for oat-based sugar-free muesli-type cereals, unsweetened whole grain cereals, porridge oats, corn grits, Maltabella (malted sorghum porridge).
   c. Change white flour in any recipe for whole grain flour (if you take whole wheat flour and want to make a cake then sift it, add back half the bran and whiz round in a blender).
   d. For thickening sauces, instead of white flour or refined cornmeal, try the same quantity of arrowroot and use unrefined coarse cornmeal for soups and chowders.

2. Increase the intake of all types of dietary fibre by changing:
   a. Animal protein for vegetable protein such as mycoprotein, TVP, beans and lentils, this is especially easy when making casseroles, soups and stews.

   b. Use salad or raw vegetable crudités as an Hors D'ouvres (starter) rather than a cream soup or a meat-based item such as pate.
   c. Use fresh fruit as a snack or dried fruit (too much is not recommended) to replace sweets, candies, chocolate, pastries or doughnuts.
   d. Use vegetable rather than meat-based sauces, i.e. a tomato and basil or mushroom sauce rather than gravy.

Cutting down on fats and changing the type of fats consumed can aid not only in the prevention of cardiovascular diseases [3] but also in the mitigation of cognitive decline [8,9]. The following changes may help in this respect:

1. Change the type of fat used
    a. Use olive oil for braising or basting rather than butter, lard, bacon or refined vegetable oils.
    b. Use olives or avocado pear in a salad rather than a refined oil-based dressing or mayonnaise.
    c. If oil is to be used, then use canola oil or olive oil as a preference.
    d. Brush bread with olive oil, or lightly spread with a nut butter rather than using butter or margarine.
    e. Use Omega 3 rich fish rather than a fatty cut of meat.
    f. Use nuts and seeds as a snack rather than bacon bits, pork crackling, crisps, chips and pretzels (this will also cut down on salt).

2. Change the amount of fat used:
    a. Brush the bottom of a pan with olive oil and cook food covered with a lid to stir steam rather than stir-fry.
    b. Grill as opposed to frying food.
    c. Coat with whole wheat crumbs and bake foods rather than battering and deep frying.
    d. Use yoghurt rather than sour cream for toppings and tofu or quark rather than cream cheese.

e. Use vegetable-based dips such as salsa (spicy tomato and onion) and guacamole (spicy avocado) rather than mayonnaise or sour cream dips.

f. Dress vegetables with olive oil spray, or an arrowroot and lemon glaze rather than butter.

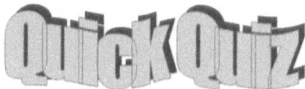

Below is a conventional recipe for a pasta dish for four people:

<u>Ingredients</u>

4 rashers smoked streaky bacon	½ cup heavy cream
3 Tbs. cooking oil	½ tsp salt
1 large onion	200 g penne pasta
1 clove garlic	2 litres boiling water
8 large mushrooms	100 g grated parmesan cheese

<u>Preparation</u>

1. Crush the garlic and salt together, finely chop the onion

2. Cut the rind off the bacon and slice crossways into strips

3. Fry the bacon, crushed garlic and onion in 2 Tbs. oil and when soft add the mushrooms, fry gently for 5-8 minutes

4. Meanwhile, place the rest of the oil and the penne into the boiling water and simmer for 12-15 minutes

5. When the bacon and mushrooms are cooked through remove from the heat and add the cream, stir gently

6. Drain the pasta and add the mushroom, bacon and cream mixture, serve with grated parmesan cheese.

We are now going to firstly look at the ingredients and make some changes:

4 rashers smoked streaky bacon   change for?   _____

3 Tbs. cooking oil   change for?   _____

1 large onion

1 clove garlic

8 large mushrooms

½ cup heavy cream   change for?   _____

½ tsp salt   change for?   _____

200 g penne   change for?   _____

2 litres boiling water

100 g grated parmesan cheese   change for?   _____

Increasing Value by Changing Cooking Methods

We looked at the subject of cooking methods and food processing briefly in learning session five, with respect to preserving vulnerable vitamins, in particular, those that are water soluble. When it comes to making the best of food, cooking methods are almost as important as the ingredients we choose, as even the best ingredients can be compromised by using cooking methods that deplete the nutritional value. In learning session five we looked at preserving the heat and water vulnerable nutrients by reducing the amount of heat, the length of time that food is exposed to heat and minimising the use of water. There are however other considerations for food preparation:

- Storage
- Bacterial contamination
- The generation of heterocyclic amines in cooked food

Storage

The fresher and closer to its source the better, as far as conservation of nutrients in foods is concerned. The main items required for the growth of cells are carbon, hydrogen, nitrogen, oxygen, sulphur and phosphorous. This applies, however, not only to human cells but to bacterial and fungi cells as well. You will notice from the inclusion of nitrogen in this list that the protein content of a food is especially important. Three other things are also important: warmth, air, a neutral pH (found most ideally in water) for growth [10]. Now, here comes the cruncher, as far as the bacteria are concerned, they are competing for the same nutrients as us, and it's an all-out 'us or them' situation. The longer the food is away from its source and the more the ideal conditions for growth, the more bacteria and fewer nutrients it is likely to contain. Left long enough there are only bacteria left and no nutrients. The only reasonable thing to do to conserve the nutrients and deprive the bacteria and fungi is to remove one or more of the conditions that they require for growth. This may be done in one of four ways, which will keep food fresher and preserve the nutrients for longer, however not indefinitely. Some are more acceptable than others, and some of these methods may inherently have problems of their own, such as salting which requires that one consumes a large amount of sodium with the food concerned.

- Removing warmth
  - Freezing at very low temperatures (-5 deg. C or less)
  - Chilling (refrigeration at between 2 and 8 deg. C). Note that cooked food fresh meats or dairy produce stored at 10 deg. C or more must be eaten within 24 hours.
- Changing the acid/alkali (pH) medium
  - Pickling in salt
  - Pickling in brine
  - Pickling in a mildly acidic solution such as vinegar or alcohol
- Removing air
  - Vacuum packing
  - Storing in sealed containers
- Removing water
  - Drying food

Bacterial Contamination

Improper storage of food, as well as inadequate cooking and poor sanitary conditions under which food is prepared, can cause serious diseases. Although many parts of the body may be infected, the gastrointestinal tract is the most vulnerable. In addition, waterborne infections may arise when water undergoes faecal contamination either from human or animal sources [10]. Norwalk viruses are those which relate to food contamination and unfortunately appear to be on the increase in the UK, and other developed countries. Known to many people as winter vomiting disease, this has recently begun to proliferate throughout the year [11]. There are some basic considerations to food preparation that one needs to bear in mind:

- Using safe sources of water for food preparation
  - Using certified tap water or filtered or bottled water for food preparation
  - Boil a small amount of water first before adding vegetables for cooking or steaming
- Washing one's hands as well as preparation surfaces and utensils before preparing food and using clean containers that have been stored with the lids on.
- Heating food as quickly and as thoroughly as possible to avoid increasing the production of bacteria and viruses and hopefully to kill off any that may be present.
  - Food should either be eaten from the fridge
  - Alternatively, if food is served at room temperature it should be either:
    - Washed, or peeled – i.e. in the case of fruit
    - Covered whilst being brought to room temperature
  - If heated, food should be thoroughly heated to above 68 deg. C to kill bacteria before consumption – never just heat the food to an edible temperature, especially if reheating previously cooked food

Heterocyclic Amines

Food processing and other culinary preparations enable food products to be made edible which not only naturally increases their appeal, but also provides stability during storage. However, some procedures are safer than others. The biggest concern is the generation of heterocyclic amines (HCAs) which have been shown to be carcinogenic (cancer causing). This problem occurs because fats can heat to higher temperatures than water, and in the process of prolonged exposure to higher temperatures the HCAs are generated. In addition, protein-rich foods seem to be particularly vulnerable to this type of chemical change with beef, pork, lamb, chicken and fish at the top of the danger list. Less problematic, unless prolonged heating in fat is used, are dairy produce, eggs, beans and peas [12].

In order of levels of HCA production, it is best to avoid the methods towards the top of the preparation list and opt for those lower down:

- High temperature roasting (160 deg. or above) of fatty cuts of meat, basted chicken and turkey and turkey covered in streaky bacon as well as anything stuffed with sausage or pork
- Deep frying foods, especially chicken and fish
- Fried bacon and other fatty meats
- Fried eggs
- Char-grilled and barbecued meats, poultry and fish
- Stir-fried lean meats, and poultry
- Dry grilled lean cuts of poultry and fish
- Stir-steam foods
- Steamed fish and chicken
- Steamed pulses, vegetables and grains
- Boiled pulses
- Foods cooked in vegetable stock such as soups and stews
- Vegetables lightly stewed in their own juices with little water or vegetable stock added

Research has shown, however, that some effects of HCA's can be reduced by the additional consumption of fermented milk products containing lactobacilli [12]. This may have been the original cultural wisdom behind the consumption of yoghurt with kebabs and fried spicy or curried meats. Perhaps if items prepared by methods near to the top of the HCA generating list are consumed on an occasional basis, then a bowl of yoghurt might be a good accompaniment.

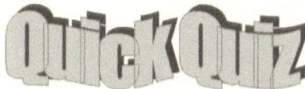

We will now go back to our pasta dish preparation. Our ingredients may now have changed, however,

4 rashers smoked streaky bacon   change for?   _____
3 Tbs. cooking oil   change for?   _____
1 large onion
1 clove garlic
8 large mushrooms
½ cup heavy cream   change for?   _____
½ tsp salt   change for?   _____
200 g penne   change for?   _____
2 litres boiling water
100 g grated parmesan cheese   change for?   _____

How would you now like to prepare this dish?

<u>New Preparation Instructions</u>

1. _____

2. _____

3. _____

4. _____

5. _____

6. _____

7. Serve with: _____

_____

Building Recipes from Your Own Dietary Plan

Traditionally, people in Westernised countries have built recipes and menus around the protein component of the meal. This has meant thinking first about the meat, poultry or fish you are going to eat and planning other ingredients around it. In the UK, chicken and turkey are consumed by the largest numbers of the population, followed by bacon, ham, beef, veal and pork [13]. In the Mediterranean countries, the grain part of the meal has been considered first, i.e. pasta; couscous; bread such as pita, or flatbread. In Asian and African countries, the grain has also been the first item in one's mind this being cornmeal, millet, or rice, alternatively, cassava, yams, or sweet potatoes [14].

Globally, there is an increase in the amount of meat, sugar and refined starches being consumed as well as refined fats and oils, while the amount of wholegrain products, fruits and vegetables consumed, is declining. This is especially obvious in the Americas and Europe, however, even in middle income and developing countries the pattern of food consumption is changing [14]. In many developing and middle-income countries, hunger exists alongside the problem of dietary-induced cardiovascular disorders and obesity [15].

It makes sense to tackle the issue of nutrient density in the diet first, focussing on needs rather than deprivation and looking at requirements for disease prevention. What we are now going to ask you to do is think about the most nutrient dense foods, the fruits and vegetables and, to build your recipes around these. One cannot over consume these foods and can only benefit from consuming more than the recommended portions given in the food planning guides. After this, we can then use these recipes as central items to a meal and add on the other requirements in smaller portions. Alternatively, we can consume two or three vegetable-based dishes with a grain or tuber as it is often done in China and Japan. This ensures that one is neither going hungry nor becoming undernourished while equally ensuring that the proportions of foods eaten in each of the food groups or categories are appropriate. The following guidelines might be helpful:

- If the meal you are planning is a light meal or breakfast, think first of the number of portions of fruit that you require per day
    - o Try to place the bulk of your fruit requirement (at least two portions into this meal
    - o Add in two other items
        - ▪ 2 grains plus 1 portion of nuts, seeds or dairy/ protein/pulse

Some examples for the above might be recipes that encompass:

- Pear juice blended with banana, yoghurt and tahini
- Orange juice blended with pineapple, carrot and coconut
- Apple with apricots, oats and yoghurt (cows, goats or soy)
- Salad of apple, grapes, and melon with lemon juice and sprinkled with toasted almonds
- If the meal you are planning is a more substantial meal or is the main meal of the day, think first of the number of vegetable portions that you require in a day
    - o Try to place at least two vegetables into your recipe
    - o Add in 2 other items
        - ▪ 1 fat portion plus 1 beta-carotene / an extra fruit / pulse

Some examples might include:

- Stewed eggplant and tomato with courgettes, and fresh basil
- Salad of grated carrot and beetroot with pineapple and walnuts
- Steamed broccoli and cauliflower with new potatoes tossed in a herb and balsamic dressing
- Stir-steamed Pak Choy with celery, mushrooms and grated fresh ginger
- Cabbage and celeriac with fennel and chopped fresh herbs

Later on, we will look at completing this meal with grains, tubers and proteins.

As this session is not very long and requires a little more creativity, we have some extra time for the learning together activities.

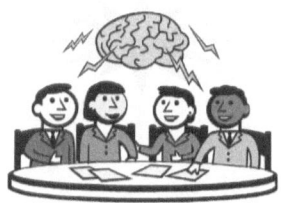

Learning Together

Learning Together

Activity 1: Allow yourselves 40 minutes for this activity

We will now have a look at building something light for breakfast, or for lunch from scratch:

Using the following different portions of foods let's see what you can come up with, in your group:

1. 2 fruits plus 1 grain portion

2. 2 fruits plus 1 grain and 1 dairy/pulse/protein

3. 3 fruits plus 1 dairy/pulse/protein

4. 2 fruits plus 2 grains and 1 dairy/pulse/protein

Now we can get a little adventurous:

5. 2 fruits plus 1 vegetable and 2 grains

6. 1 fruit plus 2 vegetables, 2 grains and 1 pulse/dairy/protein

Use any amounts of lemon or lime juice, and fresh or dried herbs or spices

Write Your Notes Here

Activity 2: Allow yourselves 30 minutes for this activity

Now we will look at building some vegetable dishes. Using the following different portions of foods let's see what you can come up with in your group:

1. 2 vegetables: 1 green and 1 other non-leafy vegetable
2. 3 vegetables: 1 green, 1 leafy and 1 other non-leafy vegetable
3. 3 vegetables: 1 green or leafy and 1 other non-leafy vegetable and one portion of food containing beta-carotene
4. 4 vegetables: 1 green, 1 leafy, 1 non-leafy and one portion containing beta-carotene

Use liberally, as you wish, lemon juice, lime juice, fresh or dried herbs and spices

Now choose 1 of the above dishes that you have created and think about what you might serve it with

Whole grains, or tubers?

Add in or serve with 1 portion of pulses/ proteins or dairy produce plus 1 fat portion

Now, what does your recipe look like?

What does your whole meal look like?

Write Your Notes Here

You may take 5 minutes to discuss your results with your facilitator if you wish

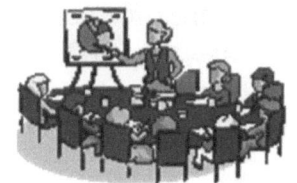

Discussion

Today's Topic for Discussion is: ARE WE EXPERIENCING THE DEATH OF THE FAMILY DINNER?

Obesity has been linked globally to both a decrease in physical activity and changes in eating habits [16]. Not the least of the latter problem, fast food outlets serving high-fat high-calorie meals are now in virtually every country, major town and city in the world. From the old-fashioned fish and chip shops, corner cafes and burger bars, to the new-fangled fusion foods, take away foods and 'ring and bring' services are fast becoming the norm for many. Previously, this was thought mainly to affect the poorer communities, especially where long hours are worked at a distance from home, and the main carer is at work most of the day. This pre-conception, however, has been disproved in a recent study which found that out-of-home food outlets are just as popular in the affluent areas as amongst the socio-economically deprived [16]. So, what has happened to the family meals? The Sunday family get-together with parents and grandparents and the dinner party society, appear to have disappeared. Is it time for a comeback and might this improve the nutritional status of society as a whole?

Some questions to think about and discuss as a group:

- How many meals do we eat per day / per week as a family on average in this group?
- What do you think prevents us from eating together more often?
- Can we think of ways to make certain meals family meals at least three times per week and then build on this habit?
- Does the same person do all the cooking in the home?

- If this person cannot for some reason cook, is the only alternative a takeaway meal?
- Do we tend to blame the fast food outlets for the way they prepare food rather than take the matter into our own hands?
- Could the cooking be shared in any way?
- Do we shy away from having visitors at mealtime, and if so why?
- Does the dinner party have to be 'posh' or can we appreciate the atmosphere created by the warmth and fellowship of others, just as much as the food?

<u>You Might Like to Make Some Notes Here</u>

References

1. Thiel RJ. Naturopathy For The 21st Century. Warsaw: Wendell W Whitman Company; 2000.
2. Earl R. Guidelines for Dietary Planning. In: Mahan LK, Escott-Stump S (eds). Krause's Food Nutrition & Diet Therapy. 11th ed. Philadelphia: Sunders, 2004.
3. Brookes L. New Dietary Advice, a New Government Program, A New Drug and a Truly Novel New BP Measurement Device. Medscape Cardiology. Volume 10, 2006:523827.
4. ADA. Evidence-Based Nutrition Principles and Recommendations for the Treatment and Prevention of Diabetes and Related Complications. Diabetes Care. 2002;25 (S1):S50-S60.
5. Food, Nutrition and the Prevention of Cancer, a Global Perspective. Washington DC: World Cancer Research Fund / American Institute for Cancer Research, 1997.
6. Yensel C, Homme DP, Curry DM. Childhood Obesity and Insulin-Resistant Syndrome. Journal of Pediatric Nursing. 2004;19(4):238-327.
7. Jensen MK, Koh-Bannergee P, Hu FB, et al. Intakes of whole grains, bran, and germ and the risk of coronary heart disease in men. The American Journal of Clinical Nutrition. 2004(80):1492-9.
8. Cassels C, Lie D. Major Cognitive Decline Linked to High Fat, High Copper Diet. Medscape Medical News. 2006(542990).
9. Crawford MA. The role of dietary fatty acids in biology; their place in the evolution of the human brain. Nutrition Reviews. 1992(50):3.
10. Pelczar MJ, Chan E, Krieg NR. Microbiology Concepts and Applications. New York: McGraw-Hill; 1993.
11. Lopman A, Reacher M, Gallimore C, Adak G, Gray J, Brown D. A summertime peak of "winter vomiting disease". Surveillance of noroviruses in England and Wales 1995-2002. Biomed Central Ltd Public Health. 2003;3(13).

12. Robbna-Barnat S, Rabache M, Rialland E. Heterocyclic Amines: Occurrence and Prevention in Cooked Food. Environmental Health Perspectives. 1996;104(3):280-8.
13. The National Diet and Nutrition Survey: Adults aged 19-64 years. London: Food Standards Agency, 2002.
14. WHO. Obesity: preventing and managing the global epidemic. Geneva: World Health Organisation, 1998.
15. Reddy KS, Yusuf S. Emerging Epidemic of Cardiovascular Disease in Developing Countries. Circulation. 1998; 97:596-601.
16. Macintyre S, McKay L, Cummins S, Burns C. Out-of-home food outlets and area deprivation: case study in Glasgow, UK. International Journal of Behavioural Nutrition and Physical Activity. Volume 2, 2005.

LEARNING SESSION TWELVE: MENU PLANNING AND SHOPPING LISTS

Introduction

Putting together menu plans is the focus of this session. We look at planning menus from your own recipes that fit in with your own dietary programme. We also look at what to do about family menus and menus that will suit you as well as others that you might be caring and cooking for. We move on next to looking at seasonal recipes, seasonal celebrations and menus to match the local availability of fresh foods.

We learn how to create shopping lists to match the seasonal purchases and standard lists for the year that can be used for the changes in climate and the availability of local produce. We look at how to create standard food orders and planning your shopping to a budget as well as the constraints one might have such as time and equipment as well as convenience and distance from the places where you shop. Finally, we discuss how constraints can be overcome in a practical manner and the advantages and considerations of shopping for food online. The quick quizzes in this learning session will help us get to grips with the practicalities of putting what we know into action and making up menus and shopping lists.

In the learning together sessions, we take an objective look at menu planning practicalities as well as the near Olympic sport of spending money and pool suggestions and helpful hints that might reduce the outgoings, and / or improve the quality of purchases. Finally, in the discussion session, we take a long hard look at how we can better take control of our choices and purchasing power to our own rather than someone else's benefit. We ask about the power of persuasion: are we being sold to, or sold out?

Planning Menus from Your Own Recipes

The first step toward the prevention of disease is the acceptance that many diseases are largely preventable through diet. The second step moves from acceptance to action [1]. To a large extent, we have already done this together by looking at our individual needs and planning our own dietary programme, daily and weekly intake of foods. Now we come to planning our weekly menus. This involves going back to our weekly dietary plan and looking at our needs in a slightly different light.

We can look at the portions of different food groups, exchanges or categories that we require and think of the different foods that might be appropriate in each. In the grain and cereal category there are many items that can be used to fulfil our requirements, for instance:

- Rice
  - Whole long grain rice
  - Brown Basmati rice
  - Arborio rice
  - Chinese black or green rice
  - Rice cakes
- Wheat
  - Whole wheat bread
  - Whole wheat pasta
  - Spinach pasta
- Oats
  - Porridge
  - Muesli
  - Oatcakes
- Maize
  - Polenta
  - Tortillas
  - Corn cakes
  - Porridge

There are many more than this, and we will shortly take another look at our choices.

In any good dietary plan, one requires variety [1-3] and the more variety in the diet, the more likely it is that one will obtain all the required nutrients without having to resort to supplements or special foods or formulations [3-5]. We now go back to our original weekly plan and begin to see not only which types of foods we require as far as groups of foods are concerned but how many different foods come into each category. What we now do is pretend that we have in fact bought all those portions of food, multiplied by the number of people in our family of course. Chefs in exclusive restaurants do this all the time; the menu changes according to availability.

Our basic recipes, as we have seen, are not fixed but can be changed according to improvements, requirements and availability. The secret is to build or adjust recipes according to one's new food list and try to use all the required foods for the week. As some items in our list become 'used up' we naturally work with what we have left, and the daily menu naturally varies. Planning menus in this way avoids certain problems, not the least of them what to eat at the end of the week and, the day before shopping day, Spartan dinner.

Recipes, as we have seen, combine various ingredients and can be made up from different foods in a single category, or several items from more than one category. With recipes, it is important to put foods that complement each other together, but they do not necessarily need to fulfil nutritional requirements in themselves. Menus are however different in this respect. A single meal should ideally contain some carbohydrate-rich foods, some protein-rich foods, some vitamin and mineral rich foods and perhaps a fat rich food. The day should contain as much variety and as many of the different food categories as possible.

The whole idea of planning food for a week is so that, overall, one day of compromise can be compensated for by another day of increased variety and nutritional content. This means that we can balance the diet over a longer period, making it less rigid. It also means that we do not have to worry so much if we are invited out or go to a restaurant, we can compensate for anything we have had too little or too much of in the days that follow.

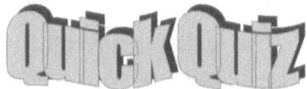

We are now going to look at choices of individual foods and experience between us the variety of foods that might be contained in any given food group:

1. Circle in red the protein-rich foods:
2. Circle in yellow the tubers
3. Circle in orange the beta carotene-rich foods (these may be fruits or vegetables)
4. Circle in brown the pulses
5. Circle in green the green and leafy green vegetables
6. Circle in blue the fruits

(NB: Some foods will have more than one circle around them)

Salmon   Sweet Potatoes   Chickpeas   Pak Choy

Blueberries   Calabrese   Mung beans

Mackerel Gem Squash Lentils New Potatoes   Pumpkin

Broad beans   Cauliflower   Pomegranates

Okra   Adzuki beans   Cantaloupe   Jerusalem artichokes

Mackerel   Gem Squash   Lentils

Endives   Loganberries   Peas   Nectarines   Eggs

Navy beans   Kale   Mange Tout   Globe artichokes

How many of the above items have you not heard, of or used yourself? Does anyone in your group know what to do with these? Take a few minutes to discuss them.

You can be creative with a day's menu planning you do not have to stick to the traditional three meals per day. Look instead at some of the following daily options:

- Two moderate-sized meals and two large snacks
- Six large snacks
- Four moderate-sized meals
- One meal and five small snacks
- Two meals and four small snacks

Research shows that the more frequently you eat, the better your digestive system functions as both peristalsis and the flow of digestive enzymes are maintained [6]. In addition, there is no law that states that breakfast must consist of cereal and milk, pastry and coffee or toast and tea. You can be creative with anything from a light fruit smoothie, to a tuna salad sandwich. This is your life and your nutritional programme. The steps to menu planning are:

1. Look at your needs for a week and add to this basic plan the special requirements that others in your household may have.
2. Divide each of your days into 'eating experiences', these may be meals or snacks that make up roughly the day's requirements and complete together the week's requirements. Now slot in your recipes.
3. Look at what is left over of your food group requirements and then add to this basic list the needs of others if they are different. Incorporate as much variety as possible.
4. Form these into meals and snacks (you can borrow from another day's allowance if your weekly needs are met). The more smaller meals you have, or the more courses one has in the main meal, the easier it is to accommodate different requirements in a given household.
5. Try never to eat less than three times per day, between three and six times per day is ideal.
6. You can use different eating patterns throughout the week if this suits social, travel and work arrangements, e.g. four meals one day and six snacks on another day.

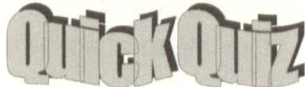

Let us look at weekly meal plans for a single person in this exercise and see how we can add variety and fill in the chosen food groups on your chosen plan by filling in the gaps:

	7.00 am	10.00 am	2.00 pm	7.00 pm
Monday	fruit smoothie	whole-wheat salad sandwich	?	wholegrain pasta with vegetables
Tuesday	fruit and yoghurt	?	large mixed salad	?
Wednesday	?	whole grain bagel with cream cheese and cucumber	?	grilled fish with new potatoes and vegetables
Thursday	fruit smoothie	?	humus salad sandwich	Basmati rice with lentil and vegetable curry
Friday	?	?	meeting friends at Tapas bar	?
Saturday	fresh fruit platter with cottage cheese	?	Large mixed salad	going out to a Chinese restaurant
Sunday	?	grilled tomatoes and mushrooms with toast	roast chicken dinner with vegetables potatoes and gravy	?

Rotating Menus and Eating in Season

If one went back fifty years, foods that were not seasonal and local were generally not eaten, for no other reason than the fact that they were not available unless imported and importing foods was more expensive. This is no longer the case and often foods, such as strawberries and avocado pears, are available all year round. The question is whether we should be eating such foods all year round. The more naturopathic view is that we were built physiologically to eat what is around us, grown locally and was provided by nature to coincide with seasons and requirements. An example would be the use of fresh spring greens in salads and light broths for the warmer weather, which was purported to thin down the blood and make one less prone to heat.

There is some scientific value in that such foods are high in potassium which has been found to lower blood pressure, in the process making one less prone to overheating [7]. In the autumn, the traditional harvest is rich in fruits and squashes, providing an abundance of the antioxidant nutrients that would build resistance to diseases during the winter months [8,9].

Eating in season might make some sense from a health perspective, but it also makes sense from an ecological and economical expense as local, seasonal food is less likely to be expensive, more likely to be available and does not require transportation over large distances. It is also good over the long term to ring the changes nutritionally to have a larger variety of food intake without going to great expense. Incorporating seasonal variety into a menu makes it easier to come up with recipes and menu plans that change, three or four times per year, maintaining variety throughout the year. Over the longer term, small differences and deficiencies in micronutrient intake are compensated for. In temperate countries, there will be four seasons and four menu changes during the year and in tropical countries, three. The secret to seasonal menu planning is to maintain priorities about eating that do not compromise overall nutrition but utilise the best of what is available, without going to extraordinary lengths.

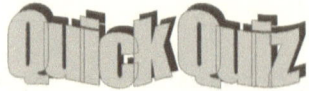

Let us look at some of the different types of foods that are seasonal. The main foods that have seasonal availability are those that we eat fresh, the fruits and vegetables.

If you are living in a temperate zone, think of some fruits and vegetables that you might use in the various seasons, given below. If you live in a sub-tropical or tropical area look at the three seasons that follow.

Temperate Zone

Spring   **Summer**

FRUITS	VEGETABLES	FRUITS	VEGETABLES

Autumn   **Winter**

FRUITS	VEGETABLES	FRUITS	VEGETABLES

Tropical Zone

Hot   **Cool/Dry**

FRUITS	VEGETABLES	FRUITS	VEGETABLES

Rainy/Storm/Monsoon

FRUITS	VEGETABLES

Shopping Lists: Save Time Money and Problems

Food choices are influenced by many factors: culture, nutritional requirements, economics and resources as well as the ability to prepare food s[3]. On top of this, we have the law of supply and demand. Given enough interesting options, youngsters began to choose lower fat items on school menus once they became consistently available. Over a two year period, the lower fat items won out over other foods due to increasing popularity and demand [10]. Research has found that students who had access to full meals which contained fruits and vegetables consistently consumed two portions of fruits and vegetables per meal as opposed to those who only had a snack bar and fast food options [11,12].

Where food choices in the marketplace are limited, there is a tendency to cater to the perception of what people want rather than the reality of what people want. Shops and stores may sell limited numbers of foods, or foods of a specific type only, rather than broadening out the availability of items [13]. This can create a vicious circle of simply eating what is available rather than making demands. Marketing is not a one-way street. Research has shown that when food choices widen through demand, there is also an equivalent knock-on effect and, when a plentiful supply of fresh fruits, vegetables and other healthy food choices are available, then these items are, in fact, bought and eaten [14].

There are two main drivers of the marketplace; one is the demand and supply chain, the other is the cost-effectiveness factor. In the first instance, making a shopping list has two purposes. The main purpose is that you have a clear idea of what you want which you have drawn up from your needs. The second purpose is that the supplier knows what you need, and you become a participant in the chain of demand and supply rather than a victim of it. When an item is demanded often enough for long enough, it is supplied. One has to make one's requirement known and learn to be assertive about having one's nutritional needs met.

The second consideration of cost-effectiveness is equally important in the marketplace and will impact heavily on public demand and the supply. Items heavily in demand can often be sold at far lower prices than an equivalent item which is required only by a small niche market. Superficially, diets high in fats and sweets and lower in fruits and vegetables have the immediate effect of costing less per calorie overall, though the quality of such diets was equally low. Costs of meat-free diets tended to be considerably lower, with meats being the most expensive items purchased. Grains and dairy produce neither increased not decreased the cost of the food bill overall as these items were priced similarly regardless of whether or not the healthier options were chosen [15]. When considered alongside the cost of lost work days, medical appointments, prescriptions, dentistry and over the counter palliatives for ill-health, the saving on cheaper food options is very short-term and temporary.

Making up our shopping lists from your nutrition plan is quite simple, one first goes back to the weekly reminder sheet for the plan one has chosen, then the following applies:

1. Add on to the requirements of the weekly nutrition plan for yourself those of other members of the household.
2. Divide the portions of each food group into portions of different types of foods.
   a. For the fruit group, for instance, you might require in total 100 portions of fruit for the household
   b. In the Autumn season, this might translate into 15 apples, 15 pears, 1 kg red grapes, 1 kg greengage plums, 5 nectarines, 5 peaches, 250 g blackberries, 250 g mulberries, 250 g raspberries, 1 large melon, 2 lit cranberry juice.
3. Try to incorporate as much variety as possible whilst retaining as many items as possible that are local to your area and seasonally available.
4. Add in any items such as herbs and spices, as well as lemon juice, lime juice and other seasonings that you may require.

5. If you follow steps 2 and 3 for each of the food groups, you can compile a basic seasonal shopping list.
6. You will now be left with three or four lists incorporating everything your household requires to eat.

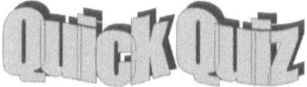

Now follow steps 2-3 above for vegetables (and if you are working with the colour wheel the beta carotene-rich foods). To help you are the guidelines and a list of seasonal foods [16].

1. Take your own weekly portions of vegetables   _____
2. Add on the portions required by others in your home   _____
       Total   _____

3. Now, divide your total number of portions by 5 and try to find food for each five portions.
4. Formulate a shopping list of vegetables with at least 5 different varieties, choosing from those below:

_____   _____
_____   _____
_____   _____
_____   _____
_____   _____

Winter / cool, dry seasons:

Beetroot, cabbage, cauliflower, celeriac, chicory, kohlrabi, leeks, parsnips, spinach, sprouts, swede, turnips, shallots, winter squashes

Spring / early rainy season:

Asparagus, broccoli, cabbage, cauliflower, carrots, courgettes, lettuce, morel mushrooms, peas, peppers, radishes, kale, mint, parsley, rosemary flowers, spinach, tomatoes, watercress

Summer / late rainy season /hot season

Asparagus, aubergine, cabbage, carrots, cauliflower, celery, fennel, French beans, lettuce, mange tout, oyster mushrooms, spinach, sweet corn, tomatoes, watercress

Autumn

Aubergines, basil, beetroot, carrots, courgettes, cucumber, French beans, mushrooms, onions, parsnips, plum tomatoes, spinach, sweet corn

You are not alone in your quest for better food. Although it may seem that we are swamped by the marketing campaigns of global organisations and food producers, there is an ongoing campaign from the 'health and well-being corner' that is gradually gaining a foothold. Project LEAN is an ongoing national marketing campaign that has been launched by the American Dietetic Association that has three goals for national campaign strategies [17]:

- To accelerate the trend to reduce dietary fat consumption from current levels (37%) to less than 30%
- To increase availability and accessibility of low-fat foods in supermarkets, restaurants, cafeterias, schools and vending machines
- To promote collaboration between national organisations and community organisations around low-fat messages and programme strategies

Budgeting for Food

Food is that with which we nourish ourselves, gain energy and prevent disease. It provides the basis of our health, and without health, we cannot work, earn, or enjoy our lives. Budgeting for food is not easy when one has many items to budget for, it is, however, based partly on priorities and partly on information. When we know why we are doing what we are doing the motivation to provide for our needs give us scope to re-plan how we manage our finances. This might mean cutting back on other items such as alcohol and non-nutritious foods and snacks in order to have available funds for the food items we really require [18]. There are ways to save; however, other tips for shopping that also help you to keep to the list that you have chosen include:

1. Avoid food in pre-packs and bags if possible
   a. This reduces cost and wastage
   b. You get to choose by hand the fruits and vegetables you want
2. Avoid taking small children shopping
   a. Swap caring duties with another parent or family so that you and they can shop in peace without the influence of 'child height marketers'
3. Avoid buying unplanned items
   a. This helps to keep to a budget and avoids impulse buying of unhealthy items
4. Eat just before you shop
   a. If you are not hungry, you are less likely to buy snack items or over purchase on quantities
5. Stick to your list as far as possible

Other ways to save time and money are to use the growing plethora of shopping services. Local shop and drop services call at several small shops with your shopping list and usually charge 3% of the total amount for the service including delivery. On-line shopping has now extended to superstores and gives you the opportunity to create and store both basic and seasonal shopping lists for delivery. Times for delivery often include out of normal office hours and weekends. Other options include emailing a shopping list for collection and payment at designated times. Having others choose your food can have both advantages and considerations, some of these are given here:

Advantages:

- You order your food according to your plan and are not influenced by other items available

- You know before you make your purchase and approve payment exactly what the cost will be and can keep within your budget or adjust your budget to your food requirements
- This may be time-saving as you can do other things at home such as cleaning, washing or child minding whilst your food is picked and delivered to you
- If something is not available, you are given the nearest option which you can accept or refuse
- The delivery cost may well be less than what you would have paid for petrol and parking; there is also a carbon emission saving!
- You do not have to be close to a superstore, take buses, mini-taxis or carry bags, this means you can get the items you need even at a distance.

Considerations:

- Someone else is selecting your items for you, and a certain amount of trust is required in their doing their job to the best of their ability.
- You may have to return items with the delivery person if you do not want them, some people find this difficult, especially if they are not a particularly assertive person.
- Setting up an account online and inputting the information your seasonal shopping lists is initially time-consuming and one requires some computer know-how or help from someone who has some experience.
- If you prefer the social contact of shopping or look forward to a day in town, this method of buying groceries may not be for you.

Overcoming Other Resource Challenges

Besides budgets and distance from shops, other resource challenges include kitchen equipment, power supplies and know how. Despite the plethora of equipment and complicated cooking procedures displayed on TV programmes and in cookery books, it is not necessary to go to celebrity chef lengths to put together a healthy meal. The less done to food, the more likely it will retain its nutritional value, the better the results. Even if one is living in a single room (the author has in fact done this, while at university), the only equipment that one really needs to cook is a plug-in electrical three tier steamer. Steamers steam vegetables, rice and potatoes, stew fruit and steam fish, adequately as well as making a good job of re-warming food. Most will come equipped with a rice cooker, and cooking bags, foil or lightweight containers can be used for fish.

If power supplies are intermittent, then a bottled gas ring stove, barbecue, or camping stove might come in handy for occasional use, when the power lines are down, as frequently happens during the storm season. A steamer insert in a pot of water can be used for a mixed vegetable dish or have some single pot casserole recipes handy that combine vegetables and pulses and can be eaten with wholegrain bread. Floating candles in a water-filled glass bowl lined with tin foil will enhance the light from the candles if there is no electricity available at all.

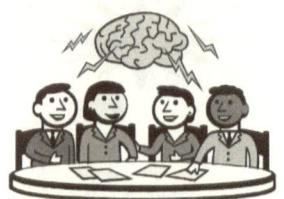

Learning Together
Learning Together

Activity 1: Allow yourselves 20 minutes for this activity

As a group fill in the meals and snacks and see how together, you can fill the gaps in the menu with the food requirements left over:

	7.00 am	11.00 am	2.00 pm	7.00 pm	Total
Monday	Fruit Smoothie	Wholegrain toast with a poached egg	mixed salad, olives whole grain roll		2 fruits 4 grains 2 green veg 1 carotene 1 ω9 fat 1 protein
Tuesday	Fresh fruit platter	Muesli, Yoghurt		Grilled salmon, steamed vegetables, new potatoes	3 fruits 2 grains 1 ω6 fat 3 proteins 2 green veg 1 carotene 1 pulse 2 tubers
Wednesday	Fruit and yoghurt smoothie		mixed salad, 4 oatcakes		2 fruits 1 protein 2 green veg 1 carotene 1 ω6 fat 2 grains
Thursday	Fresh fruit platter	Muesli Yoghurt			3 fruits 2 grains 1 ω6 fat 1 pulse

Friday	Fruit smoothie		mixed salad, whole grain roll with hummus		2 fruits 2 green veg 1 carotene 2 grains 1 pulse
Saturday	Fresh fruit platter	Muesli, Yoghurt			3 fruits 2 grains 1 ꞷ6 fat 1 pulse
Sunday	Sleep!		Quorn roast with baked potato and 3 steamed vegetables, mushroom sauce	Vegetable soup and wholegrain roll with humus pickles, radishes	3 proteins 2 tubers 6 greens 1 carotene 1 pulse

Missing Portions

7 fruit

40 grains

10 tubers

10 pulses

9 beta carotenes

21 green vegetables

5 proteins

6 ꞷ9 fats

14 ꞷ3 fats

4 ꞷ6 fats

Write Your Notes Here

Activity 2: Allow yourselves 30 minutes for this activity

The BIG FANTASY SHOP – below are shelf items and prices in a supermarket, this could be actual or online, it really makes no difference (remember that this is a fantasy shop and the prices may or may not be realistic). The game plan is that, between you, you can make up as near to ideal as possible, a shopping trolley that contains items from all the nutritional food groups for a family of two adults and two children, for two weeks or longer. You have R 1,500 (100 US$ / £85.00) to spend as wisely as possible.

Here are the shelves: R/$/£   R/$/£

Fruits and Vegetables:

Bananas 1 kg	11.20/0.75/0.65	Green beans 1 kg	19.80/1.35/1.10
Apples 1 kg	18.30/1.20/1.0	Pak choy x 2	32.40/2.15/1.80
Plums 1 kg	34.40/2.30/1.90	Onions 1 kg	12.90/0.85/0.72
Nectarines x 6	29.90/2.0/1.65	Carrots 1 kg	14.90/1.0/0.85
Red grapes 1 kg	38.00/2.55/2.10	Sweet potatoes 1 kg	18.90/1.25/1.0
Peaches x 6	32.00/2.15/1.75	Turnips 1 kg	23.90/1.60/1.32
Pineapple large	16.50/1.10/0.95	Courgettes 1 kg	38.90/2.60/2.15
Lettuce - large	12.90/0.85/0.75	Cabbage – large	14.90/0.95/0.85

Fridges:

Orange juice 2 lit	36.60/2.45/2.05	Mixed salad 220 g	16.00/1.05/0.85
Plain yoghurt 1 Kg	28.75/1.90/1.60	Soya drink 1 lit	18.65/1.25/1.05
Fruit yoghurt 1 Kg	35.25/2.35/1.95	Humus 150 g	24.90/1.65/1.40
Fresh milk 2 lit	24.40/1.60/1.35	Cole slaw 150 g	24.50/1.60/1.35

Dry Goods:

Brown rice 1 kg	28.80/1.90/1.60	Natural Müsli 1 kg	44.80/3.0/2.50
Easy cook rice 1 kg	18.80/1.25/1.05	Corn flakes 500 g	27.20/1.80/1.50
Canned tomatoes	10.50/0.70/0.60	Ground coffee 500 g	79.90/5.35/4.45
Canned beans	12.50/0.85/0.70	Dried peas 500 g	16.90/1.15/0.95

Condiments and Herbs:

Salad dressing	25.80/1.75/1.45	Walnut oil 250 ml	54.00/3.60/3.0
Lemon juice 500 ml	14.90/1.0/0.82	Dried herbs 50 g	16.90/1.15/0.93

Bakery:

Naan bread (2 pieces)	12.80/0.85/0.70	Rye bread 500 g	18.90/1.26/1.0
Sunflower bread 500 g	18.50/1.25/1.0	Bagels x 4 (pre-pack)	14.50/0.95/0.80

Drop your items in here ↓

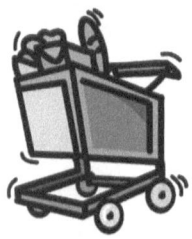

Write Your Notes Here

You may take 5-10 minutes to discuss your results with your facilitator if you wish

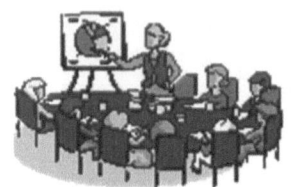

Discussion

Today's Topic for Discussion is: THE POWER OF PERSUASION, ARE WE BEING SOLD TO OR SOLD OUT?

The economically developed countries in general and the US, in particular, have produced a marvel of economic successes in the production and marketing of food, but at whose cost has this been? So far, many countries, in particular, the US have failed to regulate the aggressive ways in which food producers market high energy, low nutrient density foods. Young people are especially vulnerable and, despite the existence of a children's advertising review unit (CARU) in the US, the regulatory laws are more than 20 years old and unlikely to change in the immediate future [19]. In the developing world, the situation is also changing. The previous main causes of ill-health were undernutrition and insufficiency of calories and protein. These countries are now also experiencing the effects of global marketing, and there is a continuing increase in the consumption of foods high in refined fats and sugars. This is producing obesity and chronic diseases in a population who were often marginally malnourished in the past [20]. Young people in these countries are vulnerable as well, as they seek to emulate the British, Australian and American youth they view on TV, consuming their foods and later suffering from the same chronic illnesses [21]. Today's discussion asks: how much are we at the mercy of the power of persuasion, are we being sold to, or sold out?

Some questions to think about and discuss as a group:

- How much do you think that advertising impacts on the food your purchase, for yourselves, your families, and those you might be providing for?

- At what age do you think young people can make up their own minds about what they eat and how much influence do you think advertising has on their food choices?
- How much influence does peer pressure have on food and drink consumption and do you think that adults are just as vulnerable in this respect?
- Do you rely on advertising for information, or do you think there are enough unbiased sources of information easily available?
- It is, after all, your hard-earned money you are spending, ultimately do you think you are being 'conned' into buying things you would not ordinarily purchase if it were not for pressure, either from the media or others?

You Might Like to Make Some Notes Here

References

1. Food, Nutrition and the Prevention of Cancer, a Global Perspective. Washington DC: World Cancer Research Fund / American Institute for Cancer Research, 1997.

2. Donaldson MS. Nutrition and Cancer: A Review of the Evidence for an Anticancer Diet. Nutrition Journal. Volume 3, 2004.

3. Earl R. Guidelines for Dietary Planning. In: Mahan LK, Escott-Stump S (eds). Krause's Food Nutrition & Diet Therapy. 11th ed. Philadelphia: Saunders, 2004.

4. Franco OH, Bonneaux L, deLaet C, Peeters A, Steyerberg EW, Machenbach JP. The Polymeal: a more natural, safer and probably tastier (than the polypill) strategy to reduce cardiovascular disease by more than 75%. British Medical Journal. 2004; 329:1447-50.

5. Truswell AS. ABC of Nutrition: Some Principles. British Medical Journal. 1985; 291:1486-90.

6. Beyer PL. Digestion, Absorption, Transport and Excretion of Nutrients. In: Mahan LK, Escott-Stump S (eds). Krause's Food, Nutrition & Diet Therapy. 11th ed. Philadelphia: Saunders Elsevier, 2004.

7. Frassetto L, Morris RC, Sellmeyer DE, Todd K, Sebastian A. Diet, evolution and ageing: The pathophysiological effects of the post-agricultural inversion of potassium-to-sodium and base-to-chloride ratios in the human diet. European Journal of Nutrition. 2001;40(5):200-13.

8. Murray MT, Pizzorno JE. Beta-carotene and Other Carotenoids. In: Pizzorno JE, Murray MT (eds). Textbook of Natural Medicine. Volume 1. St Louis: Churchill Livingstone - Elsevier, 2006.

9. WHO. Diet, Nutrition and the Prevention of Chronic Diseases: Report of a Joint WHO/FAO Expert Consultation. Geneva: World Health Organisation, 2003.

10. French SA, Story M, Fulkerson JA, Hannan P. An Environmental Intervention to Promote Lower-Fat Food Choices in Secondary Schools: Outcomes of the TACOS study. American Journal of Public Health. 2004; 94:1507-12.

11. Cullen KW, Zakeri I. Fruits, Vegetables, Milk and Sweetened Beverages Consumption and Access to a la Carte / Snack Bar Meals at School. American Journal of Public Health. 2004; 94:463-7.

12. Kubik MY, Lytle LA, Hannan PJ, Perry CL, Story M. The Association of the School Food Environment with Dietary Behaviours of Young Adults. American Journal of Public Health. 2003; 93:1168-73.

13. Sloane DC, Diamant AL, Lewis LB, et al. Improving the Nutritional Resource Environment for Healthy Living Through Community-based Participatory Research. Journal of General Internal Medicine. 2003; 18:568-75.

14. Morland K, Wing S, Roux AD. The Contextual Effect of the Local Food Environment on Resident's diets: The Atherosclerosis Risk in Communities Study. American Journal of Public Health. 2002; 92:1761-7.

15. Drenowski A, Darman N, Briend A. Replacing Fats and Sweets with Vegetables and Fruits - A Question of Cost. American Journal of Public Health. 2004; 94:1555-9.

16. Seasonal Food Calendar http://sustnable.woodcraft.org.uk/1_act5a.htm. Accessed 2007 6th June 2007. Woodcraft.org.uk.

17. Samuels SE. Project LEAN - Lessons Learned from a National Social Marketing Campaign. Public Health Reports. 1993;106(1):45-53.

18. Moreira PA, Padrao PD. Educational and economic determinants of food intake in Portuguese adults: a cross-sectional survey. Biomed Central Public Health. Volume 5, 2004.

19. Kelly B. To quell obesity, who should regulate food marketing to children? Biomed Central Globalisation and Health. Volume 1, 2005.

20. Hawkes C. Uneven dietary development: linking the policies and processes of globalisation with the nutrition transition, obesity and diet-related chronic diseases. Biomed Central Globalisation and Health. Volume 2, 2006.

21. Reddy KS, Yusuf S. Emerging Epidemic of Cardiovascular Disease in Developing Countries. Circulation. 1998; 97:596-601.

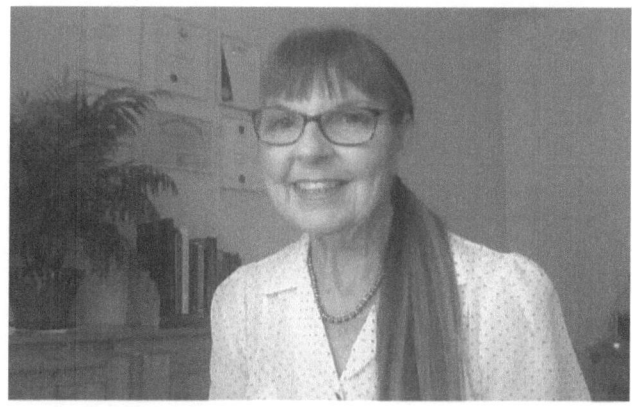

Angela Ann (Anja) Morris-Paxton

Dr Anja Morris-Paxton gained her undergraduate degree in 1986 and worked for 12 years as a nutritionist and nutrition lecturer; building nutrition education programmes for the community and for higher education institutions. She completed voluntary community service on the Island of St Helena in 1998 before moving to the UK to further her postgraduate education. Anja gained her MA (Complementary Health Studies) at the University of Exeter (with distinction) and PGCE (Higher Education) at the University of Plymouth. She worked for five years both as programme manager and as a senior lecturer with the Foundation Science programmes in the Faculty of Health and Human Sciences at Thames Valley University. After returning to South Africa Anja worked for an NGO under the WHO Civil Society Initiative, building two health education programmes (nutrition and lifestyle management). She worked at Walter Sisulu University as HOD Consumer Science and later, as Institutional Extended Programmes Coordinator, during which time Anja read for her PhD, graduating from Nelson Mandela University in April 2016. Currently Anja is a Research Associate of Nelson Mandela University and is the CEO of a research support service. She has published several papers from her doctoral thesis as well as her NGO work. This is the first set in a series of wellness education books written by this author.